THE
DUTCH
DIET

J.T. COOPER, M.D., M.P.H.

**Introduction by
Peter Van Tiel, Creator of Malsovit®**

Distributed By

LONGSTREET PRESS

**To Sarah and Bill Bedell
of Albany, Georgia,
with love and appreciation**

Distributed by
LONGSTREET PRESS, INC.
2150 Newmarket Parkway
Suite 102
Marietta, Georgia 30067

Printed in the United States of America

1st printing, 1989

Library of Congress Catalog Card Number: 89-092388

ISBN 0-929264-71-1

This book was printed by Berryville Graphics, Berryville, Virginia through Anderson, Barton, & Dalby, Inc. The text type was set in Times Roman by Typo-Repro Service, Inc., Atlanta, Georgia. Design by Laura Ellis. Cover illustration by Walt Floyd.

CONTENTS

INTRODUCTION

For many years I had been frustrated with the nutritional value of a number of the foods available on the market. As with so many people, I realized I was frustrated, voiced it to others, but never did anything about it until one night in February of 1982. Little did I know that it was going to be a memorable night which would change my life completely. That night, I was on my "soap box" again about nutrition and the lack thereof in many food products. What particularly concerned me was the fact that my children, as well as many others, were growing up eating nutritionally insufficient foods. The person I was addressing was a local baker, and obviously he felt his products did not fit my description. After explaining to him that his products were also nutritionally insufficient, he challenged me to create something that would provide the proper nutrition.

Several days following this meeting, I thought about what he had told me. Rather than standing along the sideline and complaining, he told me "do something about it." My years of experience and knowledge about nutrition (besides being an avid eater) helped out. I proceeded to go to my local health food store to buy the necessary ingredients. After numerous tests at my friend's bakery, we finally produced something which looked like a loaf of bread. All I needed was about ten loaves for my family and I was set to leave. Rather than throwing the remaining loaves away (I guess we made about sixty), we called the editor of the local newspaper. The next morning an article appeared in the newspaper about a new "health bread." Many consumers responded to the article, and soon the bakery sold out. Luckily I remembered the recipe, so more batches were made. The product continued to sell, and consumers came to tell the baker how wonderful it was. The comments included reports of "feeling better," "more energetic," and "weight loss."

Once this news reached me, I re-examined the ingredients. The particular combination of ingredients would indeed help generate weight loss provided enough water was consumed along with the bread. But all that this meant was that another diet product had entered the market. Malsovit (as I decided to call the product) would only mean something to people if it would provide more than just a way to lose weight. Usually, losing the weight is not a dieter's biggest problem, but staying on the diet is. Diets usually lack variety, become boring and, along with the continuous feeling of hunger, are difficult to stay on. Those who do succeed in losing the weight (usually following a 1,000 calorie per day diet) then face the "after the weight loss nightmare" of regaining everything they lost plus some. Realizing all of this, I decided to design a diet plan that would be easy to follow, would not leave people feeling hungry and would include consumption of a variety of "regular foods" on a daily basis. The diet's maintenance phase would be designed so that people would indeed not regain the weight they lost. However, that aspect is not just a matter of "being good" after the weight loss goal has been reached. Again Malsovit's unique combination of ingredients helped me address this problem. Malsovit provides the body, on an ongoing basis, with complete protein (the essential amino acids), which prevents the body from drawing on protein in muscle tissue as an energy source. Once this happens, usually right before the so-called "plateau," the body tries to restore the protein level in the muscle tissue. To be able to restore the protein level, enough energy must be available for the body to perform its daily functions. Energy comes from what you eat (calorie is just another word for energy). Don't waste your time counting calories, just make sure you provide enough of the right kind of nutritional energy.

Earlier on, I indicated that my evening with the bakery owner was a "memorable night." Malsovit has grown over the past years and is now widely recognized by consumers as well as physicians in various fields. For those who have not tried Malsovit and therefore have never experienced Malsovit's effects, our products may be "questionable." This world is full of experts and so-called experts, and each one is entitled to his or her own opinion. For those who have tried Malsovit, there is no doubt. IT WORKS. This book is a direct result of the hands-on experiences of a doctor, whose background is in the weight loss industry. His enthusiasm for Malsovit stems from his daily successful encounters with what Malsovit has done for his patients. Happy, satisfied, slim consumers in The Netherlands, Belgium, Germany, Sweden, Norway, Denmark, England, Israel and the United States are all the testimony I need. I hope this book will help you be a better dieter. Should you have any questions, I refer you to Malsovit's toll free number (800-521-3505). Best of luck.

Peter van Tiel

CHAPTER ONE

INTRODUCING THE DUTCH DIET

This book should do more for a patient than simply tell him or her what to eat. Knowing what to eat and how much to eat is not enough. It is also important for you, the patient, to know how to deal with the factors in your life that initially lead you to develop the problem of overweight in the first place. Almost every hint or bit of information in the book will help someone who reads it, and there are enough of these nuggets of knowledge so that you should derive a lot of assistance from a great number of them.

You should start at the beginning of this book and read each chapter carefully, using a technique that seems to speed learning of this type of material. First, skim through the chapter and don't dwell on any one particular item at any great length. Next, go back after a few minutes and read each section carefully, looking for the main message in each individual part of each chapter. Lastly, wait about 20 minutes and read everything in the chapter again. This time, do any exercises or answer any questions that may appear at the chapter's end.

It is best to cover only one chapter at a time. Most will take you less than an hour to read, but don't get in a hurry and try to go too fast in covering this educational material. Give each chapter time to be absorbed and understood. If you have any questions, talk to the physician involved in your treatment. Every item of information and every bit of advice contained in this booklet has been proven to be useful and valid through personal experience of the author, or through that of a respected researcher in the field of obesity treatment. This doesn't mean that the things we ask you to do will always work for you every time, but it does mean that these actions and techniques will work for the vast majority of you who use them properly.

The Dutch Diet book is divided into a number of chapters that cover most of the things you need to know about weight loss. You will be told why most people become overweight and how continuing to stay this way can shorten lives and cause a number of serious problems in other ways. You will be instructed in how to handle situations involving your spouse, your family, your friends and neighbors, your co-workers, and others you come in contact with on a regular basis.

The inner feelings that we are not always aware of can be important in the control of problem eating. Our past experiences also affect how well we do on a weight control program. Attitudes of others toward an obese person are often quite interesting and important to know about. Overt and covert sabotage can be devastating to a slimming program, unless the person with the problem can deal with this damaging influence.

It is also important for you to realize what really happens when a pound of fat is burned by the body for energy. Important changes in what are called "body compartments" can affect what happens on the scale and sometimes discourage a dieter when he or she is really doing quite well.

The basic food groups will be covered, using a simplified way to keep track of what has been consumed and what foods are left in the daily allotment in each of seven groups. There are a lot of mistaken ideas in food choices, but the explanations given to you should correct a lot of them. If there are questions, be sure and check with your doctor to make sure that everything is clear to you. The best and most successful dieter is an informed dieter. When you are finished with this book, we hope you fit into that category.

As a former fat man of 240 pounds, I can identify with each of you who reads this book. It is not a laughing matter to be overweight, but some of my colleagues and family found my fatness amusing. Some of the doctors I consulted almost laughed in my face when I told them I was tired of being hypertensive, with high blood cholesterol and triglycerides. They were friendly, but not very sympathetic to my problems.

I finally found a group of physicians through the medical literature who were interested in overweight. The techniques that are mentioned in this book are mostly ones developed in response to their research efforts and findings. I lost my weight by using the same ideas and knowledge that you can use after you carefully read the information contained here.

HOW OBESITY CAN HURT YOU

Being overweight carries with it a significant risk for a number of problems. In addition to the decreased quality of life that an obese person has, there are now studies showing that there is increased risk from such diverse problems as coronary artery disease, hypertension and hypertensive heart disease, gallbladder disease, certain types of cancer, arthritis, respiratory diseases, traffic accidents, and strokes, to name a few of the more prominent problems.

Some risks are secondary, such as in coronary artery disease. In this condition the elevated blood pressures, increased levels of blood lipids, and problems with diminished glucose tolerance, or actual diabetes mellitus, cause the risks to be increased for heart attack and for death from this condition.

It has been observed in my practice, as well as being reported in the literature, that even modest degrees of weight loss produce marked drops in formerly hypertensive blood pressures. Part of that may be produced by sodium restriction, but a substantial amount is simply related to the drop in the fat mass of the body. Actuaries have shown that a drop in body weight produces a better life expectancy for the obese patient, in comparison to someone who remains corpulent and does nothing to help himself.

There is apparently some connection between how the fat is arranged on the body and the incidence of killing diseases, particularly heart disease. Those with a so-called "pear shape" have a lot of the fat on the thighs, buttocks, and hips. They often do resemble pears in the initial body contours prior to weight loss. Those persons with the pear shape have less likelihood of dying or being made ill from heart disease than the other, more dangerous "apple shape."

The apple person has most of the excess weight concentrated on the abdomen and has a roundness or rotundity that does resemble an apple. This second and more endangered type of body shape also may have excess fat deposits on the upper arms, the shoulders, and the area just below the neck (the dowager or buffalo hump). Apples often resemble patients with Cushing's syndrome, with ruddy faces, fat cheeks, fragile skin, poor glucose tolerance, elevated blood pressure, and pink to purple striae (stretch marks) on the abdomen and flanks.

This "Cushingoid" individual rarely tests positive for Cushing's syndrome. Any elevations in certain steroid levels are not significant when compared with surface area or weight.

Risks in men who are overweight include higher incidence of colon, rectal, and prostatic cancer. Women who are significantly overweight, particularly in certain age groups, are more prone to have cancer of the uterus (both the cervix and the endometrium, or lining), as well as cancer of the ovaries. These documented risks make it even more imperative that a weight loss program be started as soon as possible. It also means that it is important for both sexes to have proper screening for cancer, blood vessel disease, and other preventable and treatable health problems.

What can you do about cutting down on your risk while getting slimmer and healthier? See your physician for checkups at intervals decided between the two of you. Use common sense in avoiding certain "red flag" habits, such as smoking, other tobacco use, excess alcohol consumption, and general inactivity or lack of exercise of the proper type.

A good portion of the killer diseases in this country could be reduced in severity and frequency if only we did a few things a little better than we do them now. Our own mental attitudes can wreck our self-improvement efforts. We need to get motivated to do these helpful things for ourselves. Perhaps these few pages outlining the dangers will motivate, and you won't have to have your first heart attack first. Form a partnership with your doctor and his staff and make sure you don't become another statistic.

OBESITY, HOW YOU GOT IT
AND WHY IT STAYS WITH YOU

In going over literally thousands of patients over the past 20 years, I found an almost universal situation. The onset of obesity in almost all cases followed one or more stress situations. It might have been surgery, childbirth, marriage, divorce, a new job, emotional trauma, the death of a loved one, or an adult or childhood illness. Whatever happened, it was followed by a relentless and constant battle against fat gain.

The history usually shows a succession of diets, weight loss routines, attempts at exercise, and even surgery to "cure" the obesity. The story is usually the same in every case. A temporary weight loss is followed by an eventual regaining of the weight, and often a newer and higher weight after refeeding has occurred.

Medical researchers have studied the obese for centuries in order to find out why these patients are the way they are. We have found a lot of abnormalities associated with obesity, but it appears that all of these deviations from normal are the result of obesity, rather than the cause.

At one time it seemed logical to give thyroid for obesity, but this was when the testing procedures were relatively primitive and inaccurate. Now balance studies have shown that the excess weight lost while on thyroid is usually and primarily lean body tissue (especially protein) and not very much fat. It just isn't true that the glands are the cause of weight problems, except in a very small number of people. Giving thyroid without a proper test for the presence of underactivity is not considered good medicine these days. In some cases it can be possibly dangerous, but the body is fortunately very tough and can tolerate abuse such as unnecessary and unneeded thyroid.

If glands are not the problem, it must be that overweight people are gluttons. Right? Not at all. Most people with a weight problem eat less at times than their more fortunate thin friends. They tend to eat more of certain types of foods and their sense of being hungry or not being hungry is impaired.

I once was seeing an obese patient for her monthly visit and she moaned that she thought it was unfair that she had a weight problem while her friends did not. I remarked to her that life wasn't fair and probably never would be. I told her that I had to wear glasses in order to see over ten feet in front of me, while my sister had perfect vision. I explained that we have to play the hand that we are dealt and make the best of what we have. At least we are alive, although forced to diet.

I had this patient all upset because I was explaining this basic law of nature and physiology. If energy taken in equals energy expended each day, the body fat stores will usually stay the same. Whenever energy output increases over intake, we have to make up the deficit by tapping the energy in our fat stores, producing weight loss.

The opposite occurs when energy intake exceeds output. Then we can deposit a daily amount of extra energy in our fat banks, causing our fat stores to increase. The secret of all those thin people who seem to stay the same effortlessly lies in their activity pattern and the habits they have adopted of only eating when hungry.

Thin habit patterns include moving around a lot more than an overweight person does. A thin eating pattern is based mostly on internal signals. Hunger produces an episode of eating to satisfy the needs of the body. Satiety or "fullness" stops the eating, even if there is something still left on the plate. You and I are slaves to the external world when it comes to eating. We eat until the plate or bowl is empty. We also eat in response to external cues and influences. Our emotions cause us to eat as well. It is no accident that the so-called "hunger center" in the hypothalamus (a part of the brain) is quite close in location to the areas that seem to be the source of strong emotions and feelings.

What about the use of anorectic drugs, or those medications that have been called "appetite pills?" Why not just take a few of these every day and quit eating entirely? The truth is that since true hunger is extremely uncommon in the chronically obese, the use of a hunger stopper is ineffective. As it turns out, research has shown that certain of these medications do exert a positive and beneficial effect on certain cases of obesity. The indiscriminate use of them is to be condemned, however.

We can say then, that obesity is a complex condition with no easy answers, but it does not present a hopeless situation. You *do* need to know what to eat and how much. You *do* need to know how many calories are in different portions of foods and beverages. You *do* have to find some reasonable way to increase your energy output, preferably through aerobics. You *do* need to increase your sense of self-worth and gain confidence in handling yourself in food-related situations.

The most important thing is not to get discouraged or overwhelmed in this process of losing fat. The multiple things you have to deal with *can* be handled over a period of time. You have to be realistic and tolerant of initial problems and mistakes as you learn these routines that are of help to you. Look at the entire experience of losing unwanted weight as a learning experience.

In the learning process you must take tiny bits of the overall problem and deal with each one individually. Visualize a brick wall that stands between you and your goal. You obviously can't move the entire wall out of your way at one time, but you *can* tear that wall down a brick at a time. The individual "bricks" are your unique and special problems. Handle them separately. Divide and conquer! Make your experience of weight loss a pleasant one, and don't take yourself too seriously if things aren't always the way they should be.

As in any learning experience, there are lessons to be studied and homework to be done. Please look upon the extra time spent as an investment in your slimmer future. If your therapist wants you to walk, please find time to do so. If you have to go through some discomfort in order to survive at a food-related gathering, please put up with it. A long-term goal is worth some temporary problems, and the efforts you expend today will pay off dividends in health, happiness, and the chance of a longer and more productive life.

This book is dedicated to these men and women who were pioneers in the field of obesity treatment. It is particularly dedicated to the memory of Peter G. Lindner, M.D., who passed away suddenly in 1987. Peter and the other giants and path-finders in this new and exciting field of medicine were my friends and mentors. They made it possible for me, and for each of you, to reach a thinner and healthier size and weight.

I probably will never meet most of the patients who read this, but I will be pulling for each of you, along with the physician who is helping you perform this vital service for yourself. To each of you, good luck and God bless you!

The use of increased fiber in the diet of those trying to reduce their weight is not a new thing. Fiber is a healthy addition to any diet and tends to help regularity, to interfere with the absorption of certain unwanted calories and nutrients, and to give a person the comfortable feeling of fullness that is often missing in a lot of diet programs. Increased dietary fiber was also emphasized in my previous diet book efforts, including *The South American Diet*, *The Common Sense Diet*, and the *Clinic-D Program*. The last two were published by Greentree Press and are still being sold nationally.

What would have caused me to develop yet another diet book? I was content to let these exceptionally effective books be my last ones for a while, but my intentions to be inactive in a literary way were blasted to pieces by one of the most exciting, yet simple, routines I have ever come across. One of my patients told me of a diet plan developed by Peter van Tiel of the Netherlands that involved the use of SEVEN pieces of a special bread every day. This started me to thinking that someone was trying to tell fairy tales to my patients, but I decided to investigate the plan anyhow.

Mr. van Tiel had developed a bread that he named Malsovit in his test kitchen in his Netherlands hometown of Tiel. It was made from an ingenious combination of flour from a number of grains, plus bran, soy flour, and wheat germ. The finished flour product was then baked according to rigid standards set by the inventor. A loaf of Malsovit bread catches your attention immediately because of its denseness. When you pick up a loaf of it, you KNOW that you have a loaf of real bread, not just white flour puffed up with air in the baking process.

When the bread is eaten as directed, there is a sensation of fullness that develops, what my father called a "stick-to-the-ribs" feeling. The taste and texture are pleasing and the calories are only a total of 66 per slice. The fresh-baked product is moist and tasty, eliminating an often-noted feeling of deprivation that is experienced on breadless and starchless diet programs.

I still doubted that the bread was all that it was claimed to be, so I went to Hofer's German Bakery near my home in Atlanta and bought several loafs for my own "Cooper Test" of effectiveness. I was finishing a master's thesis at Emory at the time and was keeping late hours. I had my lunch on Saturday at noon — three slices of Malsovit, a salad, three ounces of turkey breast, and two large glasses of water. I began to work on my thesis and forgot about dinner. At midnight I realized that I had worked straight through without eating but was still not hungry! I actually had to make myself eat something, not because I wanted it but because I felt I should have a small meal of fruit and cottage cheese to carry me over into the next morning.

This marathon of working on a thesis had previously made me into a perpetual evening snacker, who had to carefully remind himself that diet doctors aren't supposed to overeat at night. Not with Malsovit. I was sold on it and began to try it on my patients. The hardest job I had with them was to convince them to eat all the food that they were supposed to have for each day. Each patient was supposed to eat three normal meals, plus three snacks each day. Each dieter was required to eat a total of seven slices of Malsovit daily. Not only was bread allowed, but a reasonable amount of butter, margarine, peanut butter, diet jelly or jam, or diet mayonnaise could be spread on the bread if desired.

On a recent visit to the Atlanta area, Mr. van Tiel and his sales manager spent several hours discussing Malsovit and its development to me. I was impressed by the success stories of dieters from Europe and this country who had found a reliable, safe, and effective way to lose unwanted pounds forever. I was also impressed with reports from normal weight individuals who volunteered their satisfaction with the taste, texture, and bulk-producing qualities of this unusual product. It seemed to be a perfect bread for not only the dieter but his or her family as well.

The most impressive thing about Malsovit is its combination of grain and legume proteins in the flour, producing a complete protein product for those who use it. Vegetarians and those on diets that are low in fat will appreciate the decreased likelihood of having problems with protein malnutrition. As you can tell, I was and am sold on this innovation in bakery and nutritional science. My resolve to wait a few more years before writing this book was overcome by the sheer excitement of seeing some of my patients, who were hardcore underachievers, become real life success stories right before my eyes.

I could see the unwanted pounds and the anguish of being trapped inside fat bodies both melt away, seemingly as if by magic. I know that there was no magic really, just good nutrition, but the feeling of amazement at the ease of weight loss still remains with me as I write this. What was and is true with my patients can be reality for you.

The Malsovit bread and a companion product, the Malsovit Mealwafer, should be readily available all over the country by the time you read this. If there are no bakeries in a certain area, a person may order Malsovit by calling a toll-free number that is listed in the appendix of this book.

There are no required medications, no powders to mix up, no starving or eating of unhealthy combinations of food, no ketosis, and no magic herbal combinations. You eat six times a day, usually the same foods as your family. You don't have to run ten miles a day, but a brisk walk or the equivalent is desirable for best results. In short, the entire program is common sense at its best, and it works! For those of you who have given up on ever becoming slim, read on and see how attainable your dreams of a thinner, healthier body really are.

THE DIET IN BRIEF:

BREAKFAST:
1) Three slices of Malsovit, lightly buttered, or spread with a thin coating of peanut butter (see below).
2) One egg, either boiled, or fried on a non-stick surface without grease. You may substitute ¼ cup low-fat cottage cheese, one ounce of Farmer's cheese, or one tablespoon of peanut butter for the egg. Those who must limit their cholesterol should only have two eggs a week, or use the equivalent amount of EggBeater to equal one egg.
3) One fruit selection from the permitted fruit list.
4) All the permitted beverages desired.

MIDMORNING:
1) Eight ounces skim milk, or eight ounces sugar-free nonfat yogurt, or a fruit selection, preferably not a juice, from the list of permitted fruits, or one Malsovit mealwafer.

LUNCH:
1) Two slices of Malsovit with a THIN coating of butter, mayonnaise, peanut butter, or soft margarine if spread is desired. Please don't overdo the amount of spread if used.

2) A large salad, using the permitted salad materials and dressings.

3) Three ounces, cooked weight, of lean chicken, fish, shrimp, or beef, which should be baked, boiled, broiled, charcoal grilled, pan-fried without grease or breading, or microwaved. Instead of the cooked meat selection, you may have three ounces of tuna or chicken salad, prepared with one teaspoon or less of diet mayonnaise or salad dressing.

4) All the Super Soup, lightly-steamed vegetables, or raw vegetables you want from the permitted list.

5) All the permitted beverages desired.

MIDAFTERNOON:

1) One portion of fruit from the permitted list, or eight ounces of skim milk, or eight ounces sugar-free nonfat yogurt, or one Malsovit mealwafer.

EVENING MEAL:

1) Two slices of Malsovit, prepared the same way as for lunch with a THIN coating of spread, if desired.

2) If you feel that you must have extra meat, have three ounces, cooked weight, of lean chicken, fish, shrimp, or beef. Cook the same as the lunch protein. You may have the chicken or tuna salad instead, just as you did at lunch. When possible, omit either this evening selection or the lunchtime protein and just have one portion a day.

3) All the Super Soup, lightly-steamed vegetables, or raw vegetables you want from the permitted list.

4) A large salad, using the permitted salad materials and dressings.

5) All the permitted beverages desired.

BEDTIME SNACK:

1) One portion of fruit from the permitted list, or eight ounces of skim milk, or six ounces V-8 juice, or one Malsovit mealwafer.

The Dutch Diet contains a number of different categories of food, and should be followed exactly as outlined. It is a common failing among overweight patients to "adjust" or "tinker" with a diet. The result is usually disaster and another failure. Please resist the temptation to change things. Follow the more exacting instructions that are in the next chapter. You won't be sorry you did.

Now, let's go to more detailed instruction in the next chapter.

CHAPTER TWO

THE COMPLETE DUTCH DIET

I want to emphasize something said in the last chapter. Almost the same is not good enough when it comes to choices of foods. There are a thousand traps out there for the unwary dieter, not the least of which is deceptive advertising for foods. A food may be low-fat, such as flavored yogurt, but still be too high in sugars and sodium. Other products may be advertised as being "natural" or "high fiber" or low-calorie" and still be totally unacceptable because of things in the product that the seller doesn't tell you about. The obvious answer is to be a label reader.

There is one last thing to mention before you start this program. In the initial, weight-losing stage of the Dutch Diet, there is absolutely no way that you can follow it and eat at the average fast food restaurant. The fat, sugar, and salt content of some of these foods defies belief in some cases. Avoid eating in any restaurant and *please* avoid eating someone else's cooking for the slimming phase of your program. No matter what your hostess may say, she won't cook everything the way it really should be cooked. Only YOU can do that after reading this book.

If you absolutely can't avoid eating out or going to someone's home for a meal, try having two slices of Malsovit (with or without some sort of permitted spread) and a LARGE glass of water just before going out of your home or office. Malsovit can be kept moist and fresh in a zip-lock plastic bag until eaten. This precautionary snack can often prevent a disaster in overeating. Be sure to keep it fresh as possible.

Some of my patients have taken their Malsovit to a restaurant and instructed the waiter to serve it with their salad or entree, thereby avoiding temptation from regular bread at the table.

THE SLIMMING PHASE OF YOUR PROGRAM

Approved Bread Selections

You are to have seven helpings of Malsovit bread a day. You are to eat three slices for breakfast, two for lunch, and two for the evening meal. If you are unable to eat all three slices of Malsovit at breakfast, you can carry the uneaten portion with you and have it later in the morning as a snack. Freely substituting another brand is a sure way to fail, but I am aware that occasionally you may be caught out and not be able to get the correct bread. I am also aware that occasionally you may want a change of pace in starch intake. For that reason I allow up to TWO portions a day to be other bread-like foods, but would prefer you did the substitutions as infrequently as possible.

Any of the selections below may be substituted for one or two of the Malsovit bread slices. NEVER use more than two selections from this list a day. You should have a minimum of five slices of Malsovit daily for best results. If you have two of the selections given below, omit two slices of Malsovit. If you have one selection, omit one slice of Malsovit. If it isn't listed below, it is not allowed.

Rice cakes, 2 of any type.
Roman Meal or wholegrain (wholemeal) bread, 1 slice
Any lo-cal bread (35-45 cal/slice) 2 slices
Dry bran cereal, ½ cup. Use part of the skim milk from one of your snacks for this. Don't use sugary cereals.

Malsovit Mealwafers may be freely substituted for Malsovit bread, with 1 ½ wafers equaling one slice of the baked Malsovit.These wafers have the advantage of staying fresh without refrigeration much longer than the bread. The Mealwafers are excellent to carry along with you while traveling, or at work.

Approved Spreads for Malsovit

An excessive amount of fat-containing spreads is not a good thing for your diet and will slow or stop your weight loss. A THIN layer of butter, margarine, peanut butter, or diet Mayonnaise is permitted on each slice, but you don't have to use a spread if you don't want to. The products noted below have been tested by me and found to be useful.

Peanut butter, when used, is a substitute for the egg at breakfast. It is a spread that contains fat, but it also contains a considerable amount of protein and no cholesterol. I use old-fashioned style peanut butter from a health food store when I don't make my own. Try and avoid the chunky or creamy types of peanut butter that have lots of extra things added. The older type that I prefer needs stirring before you use it but is basically just peanuts and a tiny amount of salt. It is worth the inconvenience involved to stir the natural and unhomogenized peanut butter because of the superior taste and texture you get from it.

When you use peanut butter, you are allowed *one tablespoon* a day as a substitute for the breakfast egg. The tablespoon is a level one, not a heaping tablespoon. You should only use this food as a spread once a day, and then only if you have left the egg off. You may save the breakfast peanut butter portion and use all or part of it with the Malsovit bread during the other two meals.

Margarine and butter should be of the whipped or liquid variety. Use an extremely thin coating of either one on Malsovit bread if desired. The whipped or liquid varieties don't tend to lump up and therefore tend to produce a thinner and smoother spreading effect, which can prevent a heavier caloric load of spread on the bread slices.

The following margarines are desirable to use because of their lower caloric content:

> **Blue Bonnet-Nabisco Diet Margarine**
> **Blue Bonnet-Nabisco Spread with 52% fat**
> **Fleischmann-Nabisco Diet Margarine**
> **Mazola Diet Margarine**
> **Mrs. Filbert Reduced Calorie Margarine**
> **Promise Spread Soft Margarine with 52% vegetable oil**
> **Weight Watchers Reduced Calorie Margarine**

Diet or imitation mayonnaise is also permitted if spread in an extremely thin layer on each slice of Malsovit bread. Good brands include BatterLite and Weight Watcher's. Avoid regular mayonnaise and Miracle Whip salad dressing, at least during the slimming phase of your diet program.

Approved Fruit Selection Portion List

Each of these is equal to one portion of fruit. They are all interchangeable, but it is always preferable to have the whole fruit rather than the juice. Juices are listed for those times when it is not possible to get the fruit itself, but the whole fruit, with the added fiber and bulk, plus the pleasure of chewing and the increased amount of fullness produced, makes this alternative better than the juices. As many as four portions of fruit could be consumed in a single day, depending on which snacks you choose.

The whole citrus fruit should be a large percentage of your intake, particularly when the grapefruit, orange, or tangerine is peeled and everything inside the rind but the seeds is eaten. The bioflavonoids found near the rind are important in your nutritional health and in preventive measures to keep certain problem conditions from occurring.

> **Apple, 1 small**
> **Banana, ¹/₂ small**
> **Cantaloupe, ¹/₄ melon**
> **Grapefruit, ¹/₂ small**

Grapefruit juice, 4 ounces (¹/₂ cup)
Orange, 1 small
Orange juice, 4 ounces
Peach, 1 small
Pear, 1 small
Plum, 1 small
Prune, 2 medium, unglazed
Strawberries, 1 cup
Tangerine, 1 small

For the sake of simplicity I have restricted the number of choices you have while trying to slim down. If this is not satisfactory, turn to the chapter on maintenance and select another fruit portion from the list there. Each portion in that list is equal to one fruit portion and may be freely substituted here. The only exceptions would be the syrups and granulated sugars listed there, which should be omitted during the slimming phase of your program. I had rather you not use these concentrated sweets because of their high density and tendency to make you more hungry than desirable.

Approved Low-Fat Milk Selection Portion List

With the exception of those persons not tolerant to milk products, these are the only low-fat milk products permitted. Each of those items on the list is equal to one portion of low-fat milk and is the equivalent of eight ounces of skim milk. The use of 1% milk, 2% milk, or those with higher fat content is not a good idea. You are giving up part of the fat content of the milk in order to justify the use of spreads on your Malsovit bread. Stick to skim milk where possible.

You should try and get two milk products a day, unless your doctor says use less or more. Those intolerant to milk sugar should work with a personal physician to be sure that there is an intake of adequate calcium in other fermented milk products, including yogurt and cottage cheese. Those allergic to milk itself should not use this diet unless a physician works with them in the alternate protein and calcium intake choices. This usually involves additional lean protein and oral calcium supplements, such as OsCal-500 tablets.

Buttermilk, 8 ounces, or 1 measuring cup.

Cottage cheese, 2% fat or less, 4 ounces, or ¹/₂ measuring cup.

Farmer's cheese, 1 ounce. Beware of most cheeses, they are too high in fat, at least for the reducing part of the diet.

Non-fat dry milk solids, reconstituted, 8 ounces, or 1 measuring cup.

Skim milk, 8 ounces, or 1 measuring cup.

Yogurt, from skim milk, 8 ounces or 1 measuring cup. Use Weight Watchers, or any other brand that contains 90 calories per cup. Do NOT use flavored yogurts, except as noted below, or those made with any other type of milk but skim or non-fat milk. No frozen yogurt allowed for now.

Yogurt, flavored, sugar-free and sweetened with Nutrasweet, 8 ounces. Kroger, Yoplait, and Lite n' Lively all have yogurts with from 90 to 110 calories per container. They are legal on this diet.

All other milk products and cheese are forbidden for the balance of the slimming phase of your diet program. In the maintenance phase you are allowed a relatively free choice of dairy and related foods.

Approved Meat and Meat-like Selection Portion List

Virtually all meats and related protein foods shrink by about 25% in weight when cooked. A portion of steak that weighs four ounces raw will weigh about three ounces when cooked. Avoid cold cuts and organ meats during the weight loss phase of your diet.

Do not batter and/or fry any meats. It is best to bake, broil, boil, pan-fry without grease, charcoal grill, roast, or microwave a portion. When cooking in an oven or other situations where the fat drips from the food, be sure that the meat is high enough above the drip pan to avoid coming in contact with the drippings.

All of the following lean meats are given in cooked weight portions:

Beef, 3 ounces.

Chicken, 3 ounces, with all skin and fat removed.

Fish, 3 ounces.

Soy protein, meat-like food, 4 ounces, Loma Linda or Collegedale.

Soy cheese, made with soya milk, 4 ounces.

Shrimp, 4 ounces.

Tuna, water-packed, 3 ounces. Do not use any oil-packed fish.
Turkey breast, 3 ounces.

You may have a portion of 3-4 ounces twice a day, depending on the protein food, but it would be a lot faster for you if you usually only have one. You have to decide if you want one or two portions a day.

Salad and Bulk Vegetables That Are Free Foods

For salad or munching purposes you may consume any of these vegetables in any amount, provided they are not cooked. These free vegetables include alfalfa sprouts, asparagus, bean sprouts, broccoli, Brussels sprouts, cabbage, carrots, cauliflower, celery, chard, chicory, chilies, chives, cucumber, dandelion greens, endive, escarole, kale, lettuce, mushrooms, mustard greens, okra, parsley, green and red peppers, poke, pumpkin, radishes, rhubarb, Romaine lettuce, sauerkraut (high in sodium), spinach, raw squash of all types, string beans, tomato, watercress and zucchini. Limit carrots to one daily because of the higher content of digestible carbohydrate.

You may have a large raw salad from the above list twice a day, but you can also munch on these vegetables at any time of the day, as long as they are raw or lightly steamed (stovetop or countertop, NOT in microwave) for five minutes or less. As long as they are raw or lightly steamed, you may eat unlimited amounts of them every day, virtually any time of day. Fully cooked vegetables are not allowed until the maintenance phase of your diet program. The only raw vegetable dips permitted are those with recipes listed in this chapter. Be careful of most salad dressings, which are high-calorie traps for the unwary dieter. See the list of permitted dressings in the next section.

Salad Dressings

It is obvious that no two tablespoons are the same. Except for the non-thickened, less viscous dressings, it is hard to judge just what a level tablespoon is. Be conservative and try to minimize the errors of measuring by being careful. *If the dressing isn't listed below, don't use it without checking the label first.*

No one dressing is preferred over another, but watch out for the calorie content of some of the creamier ones. A dieter who has not yet attained ideal weight should usually not use a dressing that has over eight or ten calories per level tablespoon, and not more than two tablespoons of any dressing on a single salad. You are allowed a total of 50 calories of dressing a day. The number in parenthesis following a dressing indicates its caloric content per tablespoon.

B-Lean Special Low-Calorie, No-Oil Dressing. (2)2 Calories per tablespoon. Available only in the office of a bariatric (weight control) specialist. May be used with or without added vinegar.

Herb Magic Lite Dressing — No Oil:

> **Italian dressing (4), Vinaigrette (6), or Onion Chive dressing (6)**

Featherweight Dressings:

> **Red Wine Vinegar dressing (6) and 2 Calorie Low Sodium Dressing (2)**

Good Seasons Low Calorie Italian Salad Dressing Mix. For use with water and vinegar *ONLY*. (8) NOTE — This is the only Good Seasons mix recommended.

Kraft Zesty Italian Low-Calorie Dressing (6)

Kroger Low Calorie Italian Dressing (5)

Walden Farms Reduced Calorie Dressings:

> **Bleu Cheese, Reduced Calorie (9)**
> **Classico Italian, Sodium Free (10)**
> **Classico Italian, Reduced Calorie (9)**
> **Creamy Italian, Low Fat, Reduced Calorie (35). Use carefully.**
> **French, Reduced Calorie (11)**
> **Italian, Low Fat, Low Calorie (2)**
> **Ranch, Reduced Calorie (35). Use carefully.**
> **Thousand Island, Reduced Calorie (8)**

Note — Walden Farms sells dressings by mail order when not available locally. Write them at P.O. Box 352, Linden, NJ 07036, or call them at (201) 925-9494.

Weight Watchers Dry Mix Dressings. Calories are after mixing with water:

> **Blue Cheese (20). Be careful with this one.**
> **Creamy Cucumber (12), Dill Dressing (4), French Style Dressing (10)**
> **Herb Dressing (2), Italian Dressing (6)**

Please note! Some Weight Watchers dressings are not on the list and are not permitted. Read labels carefully if not sure.

Dia-Mel (Estee) Diet Control Dressings. These come in convenient portion packets and can be carried with you in your pocket or purse. Any of this brand that has 8 calories or less per packet is fine. Read ALL labels with great care. See how many calories per tablespoon each brand has.

If your favorite diet dressing isn't on this list, feel free to read the label and see how many calories it has per tablespoon. Use this knowledge to determine whether or not it is suitable and comparable to those listed here. If you like the dressing and it is low enough in caloric content, use it.

Low-Calorie Dips

Original sources for these recipes are unknown. A total of 90 calories of dip is permitted each day. You may have less than this, but should never exceed this limit. Some of these dips may be useful as salad dressings.

Italian Creamy Dip — about 9 calories per tablespoon. Take 1 package Good Seasons or Weight Watchers *dry* low-calorie dressing mix, 1 12-ounce container low-fat cottage cheese, and 1 8-ounce container of plain unflavored low-fat yogurt. Put all ingredients into blender and blend on high speed until creamy and smooth. Chill 30 minutes before using.

Horseradish Dip — about 10 calories per tablespoon. Take 1 1/2 cups low-fat cottage cheese (Weight Watchers or similar type), 1/2 cup tomato sauce, 1 small onion (cut into at least 4 pieces), and 2 tablespoons horseradish. Put in blender or food processor and blend until smooth. Pour into bowl and fold in a 4-ounce can diced green chilies. Cover with Saran Wrap and chill for at least 30 minutes before using. Keep lots of drinking water handy.

Hidden Valley Yogurt Vegetable Dip — about 10 calories per tablespoon. Take 3/4 teaspoon Hidden Valley Original Mix, 1 cup plain low-fat yogurt, 2 teaspoons parsley, and 2 teaspoons dry onions or chives. Blend all ingredients and chill for at least an hour before using.

Hidden Valley Cottage Cheese Dip — about 15 calories per tablespoon. Take 3/4 teaspoon Hidden Valley Original Mix, 1 cup low-fat cottage cheese, 2 teaspoons parsley, and 2 teaspoons dry onions or chives. Blend cottage cheese in blender until smooth.

Add the dry ingredients and 1 teaspoon lemon juice. Blend until mixed well. Chill for at least one hour before using.

French Dip — virtually no calories. Take ½ cup tomato juice, ½ cup vinegar, ½ teaspoon dry mustard, ½ teaspoon fructose syrup or 2 envelopes dry fructose, ⅛ teaspoon garlic powder, and a pinch each of oregano, salt, and pepper. Blend all together and chill for at least 30 minutes.

Mock Sour Cream — about 13 calories per tablespoon. Take an 8-ounce carton of low-fat (½%) cottage cheese, 2 tablespoons skim milk, and 1 teaspoon lemon juice. Blend all ingredients until smooth and creamy. Use as a sour cream substitute.

Dill Dip — about 11 calories per tablespoon. Take 1 cup Mock Sour Cream, 1 minced green onion, 2 tablespoons parsley, and 1 teaspoon dillweed. Mix all ingredients in blender on low. Chill at least 30 minutes.

Mock Mayonnaise — about 10 calories per tablespoon. Take 1 cup low-fat yogurt made with skim milk (*no other kind, please!*), 2 tablespoons diet mayonnaise, ¼ teaspoon salt, and a dash of paprika. Mix on lowest blender setting, or with rotary mixer until smooth. Chill for at least 2 hours.

Buttermilk Dressing — about 16 calories per tablespoon. Take 1 cup buttermilk, ½ cup mock mayonnaise, ¼ cup sweet pickle relish, 1 tablespoon prepared mustard, 1 teaspoon salt, ¼ teaspoon garlic powder, ¼ teaspoon dillweed, ⅛ teaspoon pepper, and 2 tablespoons chopped parsley. Mix buttermilk, mock mayonnaise, relish, and mustard in bowl. Blend in remaining ingredients. Chill for at least 30 minutes.

Dr. Cooper's Super Soup

Take 2 green peppers, several whole tomatoes (fresh or canned), 5 large onions, 1 large head of cabbage, and 1 large celery bunch. Seasoning can be done with 8 beef or chicken bouillon cubes, or dry onion soup mix, along with other herbal seasonings as desired. Vary the seasoning for effect. Cut and chop all vegetables into small chunks. Boil in water with seasoning and salt and pepper to taste for at least 10 minutes. Lower heat and simmer until desired consistency of vegetables is reached. Increase or decrease water in pot while cooking to get desired thickness or thinness of soup. The soupier it is, the better, and the more filling it is. This soup may be eaten in virtually unlimited amounts before, after, and between meals, plus bedtime. You may also add other vegetables, such as mushrooms, broccoli, asparagus, cauliflower, etc. If there are certain vegetables you *don't* like, remove them from the soup and substitute another non-starchy vegetable instead.

A delicious stew can be made by taking from one to two pints of the prepared mix and placing it into a crock pot with about four ounces of chopped or sliced chicken, turkey, fish, shrimp, or other seafood. Let it cook all day with the appropriate spices and herbs so that it will be ready by the evening meal. You can also let it cook all *night* and have it ready to take to work in a thermos bottle for your lunch the next day. The meat or other protein food used in the stew is counted against the daily allotment of meat for either lunch or the evening meal. You might want to save a slice of Malsovit and have it with your soup. The combination of the two is quite filling and satisfying.

Those patients who have to restrict their salt and sodium intake can omit the canned vegetables from the soup and use fresh or frozen ones only. Bouillon cubes that are sodium-free can also be used as seasoning when appropriate. It is obvious that there is some caloric value in the soup, but it is relatively unimportant in the daily food intake calculations. Treat it as a free food.

Other Free Foods

Each of the items listed below may be used without counting them if used in the quantities noted. Individual spices are not listed, and all are permitted in the usual amounts used in cooking or food preparation.

Catsup, non-diet, 1 tablespoon daily.
Catsup, diet or imitation, 2 tablespoons daily.
Chili sauce, diet, Featherweight, 2 tablespoons daily.
Extract of almond, lemon, chocolate, or vanilla, 2 tablespoons daily.
Gelatin, unflavored. Unlimited within reasonable amounts.
Hot sauce, 2 tablespoons daily.

Molly McButter, a reasonable amount to give flavor to foods.
Mustard, any variety, 2 tablespoons daily.
Sweet'n Low liquid Butter Buds, 2 ounces daily.

Permitted Beverages

Beverages permitted include water and up to two drinks of caffeine-containing drinks (coffee, tea, sugar-free sodas) a day. Coffee and tea are drunk with a minimum of skim milk if desired, and artificial sweeteners with no calories may be used as desired. If you want to use some of your ration of skim milk for whitening your coffee, do so, but be sure and account for it. You may have up to ten envelopes of Equal or Sweet'n Low daily. Unlimited amounts of sugar-free, caffeine-free sodas, and other beverages may be had each day. Drink as much fluid as possible, but get at least 80 to 90 ounces daily. If you aren't used to this much intake, gradually raise your daily amount until you reach at least this minimal goal. Mineral water, sugar-free Kool-Aid and Crystal Light are also permitted in unlimited amounts. Avoid drinking milk, even the fat-free kind (skim and reconstituted dry milk) unless it is accounted for in the daily milk product intake. Avoid 1%, 2%, and whole milk. Avoid Gatorade because of the high sugar content. The intake of fruit juices is discouraged on the weight loss phase of this diet. We prefer for you eat the fruits themselves. Particularly bad choices are the cranberry juices and CranApple varieties, with their high content of corn syrup sweeteners. The best drink of all is water, always. Some patients drink too much of certain beverages, as I point out below.

One of the patients on Malsovit called the office and complained to us that she was extremely constipated. She had all seven slices of the bread each day, but her "high fluid intake" consisted of 20 cups of tea a day. What she failed to realize is that tea is sometimes used to treat diarrhea. When she switched to herb teas, the problem went away. Unless your doctor tells you to do something different, the best approach to fluid intake is to drink lots of water and other permitted fluids all day long. Your needs for fluids are much greater than you realize when you are either losing weight or in the Malsovit Maintenance Diet Program.

A FEW FINAL WORDS

This diet program is usually followed until the desired weight is reached. Close attention to detail will insure your success, but don't forget the maintenance program that follows in the next chapter. After getting down to a trim weight, you must KEEP it down for a relatively long time. This type of attention to followup and details of the maintenance program will help keep you from ever going back up to your old level of obesity. Read about the details of this maintenance program and kiss your excess fat good-bye for GOOD!

CHAPTER THREE

THE MALSOVIT MAINTENANCE
PROGRAM

1) Once you have reached your desired weight, you can maintain that weight loss by eating regular dinners while following the Malsovit Diet Plan for breakfast and lunch. Eat an extra slice, or have one or two Malsovit wafers, instead of snacking in the afternoon, if you feel you can't make it until dinner.

2) You must think like a thin person at all times. Never give in to fat thinking again and never give in to the saboteurs or feeders in your life. Mimic your thin friends and acquaintances in their behavior.

3) Listen to what your body says to you. Avoid false signals, particularly those covered in other parts of this book. Make sure that what you are feeling is really hunger and not just a desire for food or treats. Stress is NOT a signal to eat. Neither are fatigue, boredom, anger, anxiety, depression, sleepiness, or happiness. When the body needs food and the feeling is really hunger, then you should eat.

4) Discount a growling or rumbling stomach as a hunger signal. Also, disregard a burning or empty feeling in the upper "stomach" area. Often this is just a sign of excess acid or irritability. Food will usually stop this symptom, but so will an antacid liquid or tablet with zero calories. This excess stomach acid will often manifest itself two or three hours after a meal. There is still absorption of food from the previous meal going on in the small intestine. The body is getting food at this time and rarely needs more this soon after a meal. Keep a small amount of antacid liquid or tablets with you if this symptom is a frequent one. Neutralizing the excess acid will usually relieve the problem, without the extra and unwanted calorie intake.

5) Stay away from those people, places, activities, and foods that tend to trigger problem eating in you. Going around these problem situations is begging for trouble. Your first job is to bring your weight down to a reasonable level while remembering to continue your changes in thinking, habits, and activity while you are dieting.

6) When faced with an almost intolerable urge to eat a problem food that is not appropriate for you at that time, take the time to relax and delay your decision. Try the delay tactics mentioned in this book and let them give you the protection that they offer.

7) Try to avoid distractions while eating. Make it the only thing you do, avoiding television, reading, listening to music, and other activities that would distort or cover up your body signals. Pay attention to what you are eating and derive the maximum pleasure out of the taste, texture, and flavor of each food. Use as many senses as you can during each meal or feeding. Chew each mouthful and savor each swallow of liquid. Don't let your mouth resemble a shredder-grinder.

8) As you eat, let your senses reach inward and explore how your body is feeling during the meal. Are you getting uncomfortably full? After what seems like a reasonable amount of food to satisfy you, are you still feeling an "empty" feeling? If there is doubt, remember that it usually takes an interval of about 20 minutes between the start of ingestion of food and the feeling of fullness. Keep your eating slowed down so that the 20 minute mark is reached with some food still in front of you. If you still

are feeling truly hungry, continue your meal but at a much slower pace. The Malsovit bread will help to keep the feeling of fullness going longer after a meal is over.

9) Endeavor to eat a variety of foods. Boredom is the biggest enemy you could possibly have at this time. Make your foods tasty and interesting. Try and use your low-density foods as fillers to compliment the required foods in each group. Use soups, salads, and permitted desserts as welcome additions to your maintenance diet plan.

10) Avoid surprises and try to plan your days so that you can minimize chaos and confusion. They are the enemies of your diet and can rapidly change your success into impending failure. It is impossible to foresee all problems and difficulties, but planning can protect you most of the time.

11) Keep coming back for prescribed followup visits with your doctor. Like an alcoholic, you will harbor the tendency to regain all your weight for the balance of your life. You must carefully watch for the presence of problem foods that could enter into your daily intake pattern. In the beginning you should be extra careful and keep track of all the different categories of food consumed each day.

Your scales, measuring cup, measuring spoons, and ruler are necessary parts of your equipment on this initial phase of your program. Until you have been on maintenance for at least two months, do not fry any of your foods, except as previously instructed.

What you eat is not the most important thing about dieting, but it is important. Most of us are busy and have other things to occupy our minds during the day. It is not practical for a person on a diabetic or reducing diet to keep track of grams or ounces of each category of food.

It will not work for a vast majority of people, so over forty years ago another system was worked out that groups foods into certain categories for the purpose of keeping track of their intake.

This system was designed to let a dieter exchange different foods within the same food group as equivalent portions. Each of these different foods in the same category had about the same amount of calories, protein, carbohydrate, and fat. Since it allowed the free exchange of equivalent portions of each food group, it was called the *exchange* system. Instead of using exchanges, this book will use the term *portions* to describe these quantities of food or beverage that are listed here.

The determination of what makes up a portion or exchange can be a futile exercise in guesswork if you don't have certain tools of measurement at your disposal. The following are almost a must, at least in the initial stages while you are learning the system:

> **One or two eight-ounce measuring cups, preferably unbreakable.**
> **A set of plastic measuring spoons to measure table-spoons, teaspoons, etc. Try to find one that has fractions of teaspoons as well.**
> **A plastic ruler with inches and centimeters marked on it (washable).**
> **A small weighing scale, preferably with a weighing dish included.**
> **Optional measuring scoops that measure quarter-cup or half-cup quantities. Should be equipped with a handle.**

Get some of the glasses, cups, and bowls that you use in your home. Take the measuring tools listed above and see how much volume two, four, and eight ounces of liquid will occupy in these containers. Get some dried beans and/or rice and measure out different fractions of a measuring cup onto your own plates and saucers. See how a cup of something appears when it is on a plate. Do the same for fractions of a cup (one-fourth, one-half, three-fourths, etc.) and begin to accurately judge just how much you are really consuming. This is one of the most important exercises you will do, mostly because it gives you more and more expertise in judging portion sizes.

The last bit of judging of portions concerns the size of a portion of meat, poultry, or fish. Measurement is usually made after cooking. One good way to do this is to carefully measure out an ounce (cooked weight) of various protein foods. See how much volume it occupies by the use of the ruler. After a while it should be no problem, provided you remain objective, to visually judge without the use of a scale. An ounce of beef, lamb, pork, liver, chicken, turkey, or veal will usually measure 3 inches x 2 inches and be 1/8 inch thick.

Time and practice will usually make you experienced enough to judge the size of each type of portion in each category of foodstuff. It pays to periodically check yourself for accuracy in the measurement by using the basic measuring tools mentioned above. It may seem to be an overwhelming job, but after a month you should be a veteran at judging portions. Most people probably only eat a total of a hundred different foods during the average month. There may be certain holiday foods and beverages, but most of the time the things you consume each week aren't that numerous. Time and practice will make you an expert if you only keep working at it.

THE BASIC SEVEN FOOD GROUPS

There are six basic food groups that have to be accounted for in the weight control or weight reduction diet plans in this book. The seventh is a group of free foods that can be eaten in moderation without counting them in the total scheme of daily food intake. The basic six include fruits, bread/starch items, meat and meat-like foods, vegetables, fats, and milk products. Each of these seven groups is covered in this chapter, along with a way of keeping track of them by the use of what I call Cooper Charts. The charts are optional and may be ordered separately from Greentree Press (see Appendix for ordering information).

The food groups will be completely discussed, including what the average portion includes. We will then put the groups together in a portion-based meal plan for a day. A system of remembering the contents of each group also involves a color for each one to help with the recalling and tracking of intake during the course of a day. The logic of assigning a color to each group will become apparent as this chapter progresses.

Fruits and Fruit-like Items

Each item included in the fruit and fruit-like list contains about 15 grams of carbohydrate, usually as simple sugars, and around 60 calories for the serving or fruit size listed. For each fruit we have listed the name of the fruit or food, the size serving that equals one portion, and the number of grams of fiber per portion if this number is 0.5 gm., or more. Fruits with a C and/or A in parenthesis are good sources of one or both of these vitamins. It is a good idea to get fresh, frozen, or dried fruits when possible. Fruits canned in water, or their own juices, are permitted in moderation but are inferior in nutritive value to those that have not been through the canning process. The word syrup (even light syrup) means that sugar has been added, not a desirable situation for the person on a calorie-restricted diet program.

Certain foods mentioned in this and other groups will only be available in the United Kingdom and are included for completeness. Other fruits will only be found in certain localities during certain seasons. Their inclusion is also for the sake of a thorough coverage of the subject.

The whole fruit is always far superior to the juice, which does not contain the pulp, water-soluble fiber, and bulk of the entire fruit portion. Also, two portions of apple juice can be consumed in just a few seconds, but two apples will take many times longer to eat and will provide more satisfaction to a dieter.

NAME OF FRUIT	SIZE OF PORTION	GM. FIBER
Apple, 1 small	2″ diameter	1.1
Apple, dried	4 rings	0.7
Apple juice, unsweetened	¹/₂ cup	---
Applesauce, unsweetened	¹/₂ cup	0.7
Apricots, raw (A)	4 medium	0.8
Apricots, dry (A)	7 halves	0.7
Avocados — Not counted as a fruit — See Fat portion list.		
Banana, raw	¹/₂ of 9″ fruit	---
Banana flakes	2 rounded T.	---

Bilberries, raw	¹/₂ cup	---
Blackberries, raw	³/₄ cup	4.5
Blueberries, raw (A/C)	³/₄ cup	1.4
Boysensenberries, frozen	1 cup, unsw.	3.6
Breadfruit, raw (C)	¹/₆ small	0.9
Cantaloupe, raw (A/C)	¹/₃ of 5″ melon	0.6
Cantaloupe, chunks (A/C)	1 cup	0.6
Cherries, sweet, raw	12 cherries	---
Cherries, canned, waterpack	¹/₂ cup	---
Cranberry juice cocktail	¹/₃ cup (too much sugar)	---
Crenshaw melon	3″ wedge	0.5
Currants, all colors, raw	1 cup	2.6
Dates, dried, unglazed	2¹/₂ medium	0.5
Date "sugar"	1¹/₂ Tablespoons	---
Elderberries, raw (A/C)	¹/₂ cup	5.0
Figs, raw, 2″ across	2 figs	1.1
Figs, dried, 2″ across	1¹/₂	0.7
Fructose, granulated	1 rounded tablespoon	---
Fructose syrup	1¹/₂ tablespoons	---
Fruit cocktail, waterpack	³/₄ cup	0.9
Gooseberries, raw, sections	1 cup	2.9
Grapefruit, raw (C)	¹/₂ medium	---
Grapefruit juice, unsw.(C)	¹/₂ cup	---
Grapefruit sections (C)	¹/₂ cup	---
Grapes, small	15 grapes	0.7
Grape juice, unsw.	¹/₃ cup	---
Guava, raw (C)	1 medium guava	5.0
Haws, scarlet, raw	2¹/₂ ounces	1.5
Honeydew melon, raw (C)	¹/₈ medium melon	---
Honeydew melon, chunks (C)	1 cup chunks	---
Kiwi fruit, raw (C)	1 large kiwi	0.8
Kumquats, raw (A/C)	5 medium	4.0
Lemons, raw (C)	3 medium lemons	0.6
Lemon juice, fresh (C)	1 cup	---
Limes, raw (C)	3 medium limes	0.9
Lime juice, fresh (C)	1 cup	---
Loganberries, frz. (C)	³/₄ cup	---
Loquats, raw (A)	12 medium loquats	0.6
Lychees, raw (C)	9 medium lychees	---
Mandarin orange, wtrpk (A/C)	³/₄ cup sections	---

Mango, raw (A/C)	½ medium mango	0.8
Medlar, bletted	1 medium	3.0
Molasses, blackstrap	1 tablespoon	---
Mulberries, raw (C)	1 cup	1.3
Nectarine, raw (A)	1 nectarine 1½″ diam	0.5
Orange, raw (A/C)	1 medium, 2½″ diam	0.6
Orange juice, unsw. (C)	½ cup	---
Papayas, raw (A/C)	½ papaya or 1 cup	1.2
Passionfruit, raw	3 medium fruits	6.0
Peach, raw (A)	1 medium or 1 cup chunks	2.3
Peaches, dried (A)	2 halves	2.3
Peaches, canned, wtrpk (A)	½ cup	---
Pears, raw	½ large or 1 small	1.5
Pears, dried	1 half	1.5
Pears, canned, wtrpk	½ cup	---
Persimmon, native, raw	2 medium	---
Pineapple, raw, fresh	¾ cup	0.6
Pineapple, canned wtrpk	⅓ cup chunks	---
Pineapple juice, unsw	½ cup	---
Plum, raw, 2″ diameter	2 plums	0.8
Pomegranate, raw	½ pomegranate	---
Prunes, dried (A)	3 medium	0.5
Prune juice	⅓ cup	---
Quinces, raw	1 medium	1.6
Raisins	2 tablespoons	---
Raspberries, raw (C)	1 cup	3.7
Strawberries, raw, whole (C)	1¼ cup	1.0
Sucrose, table sugar	1½ level tablespoons	---
Tangelos, raw (C)	1½ medium tangelos	---
Tangerines, 2½″diam.(A/C)	2 tangerines	0.6
Watermelon chunks, raw (A)	1¼ cup chunks	0.6

The fruit exchange or portion is color coded orange. If you use the Cooper Chart System the reference item that has most of the commonly used fruit portions on it is also colored orange, after the fruit of the same name. When you see that no figures are given for the fiber content of a fruit portion, that omission means that we either don't know this information, or the quantity is below 0.5 grams per portion.

Fat Portion List

The foods in this category are represented by the color yellow, after the yellow of butter or margarine. Some of the foods, such as bacon, contain some protein, but it is only a small amount and can be ignored for purposes of calculating the caloric content. Each portion, or serving, of a fat contains five grams of fat and about 45 calories. This is one type of food that is highly concentrated, so we require that you take extreme care in measuring each quantity.

Many of the foods contain larger amounts of sodium and these will be marked as such. When there is insignificant sodium there will be no figure given in that column. The fats are from saturated (more solid) fatty acids and also from the unsaturated oily fats. The more liquid a fat is, the greater the proportion of unsaturated fats it contains.

FOOD NAME	SIZE OF PORTION	MG. SODIUM
Almonds, dry roasted	6 whole unsalted nuts	---
Avocado, 4″ diameter	¹/₈ avocado (Fla or Calif)	---
Bacon, fried, drained	1 slice	200
Bearnaise sauce	1 teaspoon	60
Brazil nuts, dry roasted	2 medium, unsalted nuts	---
Butter	1 teaspoon	41
Butter, sweet, unsalted	1 teaspoon	---
Caraway seeds	2 tablespoons	---
Cashews, dry roasted	1 tablespoon, unsalted nuts	---
Chitterlings, cooked	¹/₂ ounce	---
Chocolate, unsw., melted	2 teaspoons	---
Chocolate, bitter	¹/₃ ounce or ¹/₃ square	---
Coconut, shredded	2 tablespoons	29
Coffee whitener, liquid	2 tablespoons	---
Coffee whitener, powder	4 teaspoons	---
Cream (light, coffee, table)	2 tablespoons	---
Cream, sour	2 tablespoons	---
Cream, sour, substitute	1 ounce (Encore brand)	---
Cream, whipping, heavy	1 tablespoon	---
Cream cheese	1 tablespoon	---
Filberts, dry roasted	5 nuts, unsalted	---

Hazelnuts, dry roasted	5 nuts, unsalted	---
Hollandaise sauce	1 teaspoon	28
Margarine, liquid	1 teaspoon	37
Margarine, stick	1 teaspoon	41
Margarine, stick, unsalted	1 teaspoon	---
Margarine, imit., diet	1 tablespoon	46
Mayonnaise	1 teaspoon	26
Mayonnaise, red. calorie	1 tablespoon	75
Nuts, mixed or others	1 tablespoon dry roasted, unsalted nuts	---
Oil (all types)	1 teaspoon	---
Olives	10 small, 5 large (Lots of sodium)	
Peanuts, dry roasted	20 small or 10 large, unsalted	---
Pecans, dry roasted	2 whole, 4 halves, unsalted	---
Pumpkin seeds, dry roasted	2 teaspoons, unsalted	---
Salad dressing, mayo type	2 teaspoons	100
Salad dressing, mayo,diet	1 tablespoon	100
Salad dressing, all types	1 tablespoon	---
Salad dressing, reduced calories — See Free Foods Group.		
Salt pork	1/4 ounce cube heavy sodium content	---
Seeds, dry roasted, no shells	1 tablespoon, unsalted	---
Tartar sauce	1 teaspoon	60
Walnuts, dry roasted	2 whole, unsalted	---

A diet that is low in fat is usually perceived as somewhat "dry" and unpalatable to anyone on it. The addition of small amounts of fat into the daily intake does a lot to make the foods more pleasant to consume. These are dense foods, with a lot of calories concentrated into a small volume. They must be carefully measured and used to avoid getting too many calories each day.

A bonus in fat portions may be obtained by using nonfat and low-fat milk products instead of whole milk that contains 3¹/₄% butterfat, or milk products made with whole milk. This bonus in extra butter, mayonnaise, or other fats is not given for using meat products that are lower in fat. The method for determining the fat content is given in the milk and meat products sections.

Milk Products Portion List

This group consists of milk with varying amounts of fat content and also products made from milk with different amounts of fat. If yogurt or cheese is made from whole milk, the fat content stays the same. Only the lactose is destroyed by fermentation, with the fat remaining to contribute the same amount of extra calories as before.

Regular whole milk can have almost 4% fat, or as little as 3¹/₄% in content. For simplicity, we will round off the content to 4% for purposes of figuring out the bonus fat portions that can be earned for using milk products with a lower fat content. Skim and very low-fat milk has almost no fat and will be marked with a double asterisk (**) to signify a bonus of two fat portions for every milk portion used with this amount of fat.

Low-fat milk has about 2% fat and is marked with a single asterisk (*). For every portion of this type of milk, add one fat portion as a bonus. Milk products with no marking have the full fat content and have no extra fat allowed as a bonus.

Milk has a white color code when the charts are used to keep up with what is consumed, corresponding to the color of milk. If you use a whole milk product with no asterisk there is no fat bonus. If the milk product has a single asterisk, add an extra yellow portion to your daily intake chart for each moderate-fat milk portion used. If there are two asterisks by a milk product, you may have two extra yellow fat portions for that day.

The approximate cholesterol and sodium content of each portion are listed in the following table. Portion sizes vary according to a person's measuring ability, so these figures are approximate only. MGC in the table refers to the milligrams cholesterol per serving. MGS refers to the milligrams of sodium per serving.

The latest exchange or portion tables tend to group cheeses, including cottage cheese, as meat-like foods. They are in those tables and count as major protein sources but still are good sources of calcium.

FOOD NAME	PORTION SIZE	MGC	MGS
Buttermilk from skim**	1 cup	7.8	280
Buttermilk from 2% *	1 cup	9.0	257
Butter — Not considered a milk portion — See Fat Portion List.			
Cheese — Usually considered with the meat-like foods — See Meat-Protein List.			
Coffee whitener — See Fat Portion List.			
Cottage cheese — See Meat-Protein List.			
Cream — See Fat Portion List.			
Cream cheese — See Fat Portion List.			
Evaporated milk, skim**	¹/₂ cup	4.0	148
Evaporated milk, whole	¹/₂ cup	37.0	133
Goat's milk, 4.5% fat	1 cup	28.0	122
Margarine — See Fat Portion List.			
Nonfat milk, dry**	¹/₃ cup	5.0	145
Nonfat milk, mixed**	1 cup	5.0	145
Milk, skim**	1 cup	4.0	126
Milk, ¹/₂%**	1 cup	7.0	123
Milk, 1%*	1 cup	10.0	123
Milk, 2%*	1 cup	18.0	122
Milk, whole	1 cup	35.0	119
Soybean milk*	1 cup	----	55
Soybean milk-Soyamel	1 cup	----	190
Tofu-based frozen desserts — Avoid usually. Has added sugars.			
Yogurt, plain nonfat**	¹/₂ cup	7.0	80
Yogurt, plain, added nonfat milk solids*	¹/₂ cup	2.0	87

Yogurt, flavored — Only use those sweetened with Nutrasweet. One portion containing 90 to 110 calories is allowed. Use only Kroger, Lite N' Lively, and Yoplait.

Yogurt, frozen — Avoid usually. Also has added sugars.

Vegetable Portion List

Some of the foods traditionally thought of as vegetables are higher in starch content and are usually grouped with the bread and starchy category. This would include root vegetables (potatoes, yams, etc.) and those seed vegetables that have higher starch content (corn, peas, beans, etc.). A good rule, but one that has exceptions listed, is to think of foods derived from the stems, leaves, or pods of a plant as vegetable foods. When we use the Cooper Charts, we usually use green as the color code for vegetables, as opposed to brown for the bread-starch group.

Canned vegetables tend to have higher sodium content. Certain vegetables are high in sodium in any state, including raw. These are marked in the food lists. Vegetables high in vitamin A and/or C are marked as we did in the fruit list. Those vegetables that have almost no available calories when eaten raw are marked with an asterisk (*) as a free food. They may usually be eaten in reasonable quantities and not accounted for if they are either raw, or steamed for less than five minutes.

If the vegetable, whether marked or not, is steamed for longer than five minutes or cooked completely, it counts as a vegetable portion and is no longer a free food. The cooking process, if done long enough, breaks down the cellulose and other complex carbohydrates into a digestible, and therefore accountable, food with usable calories for the body. Some vegetables are rarely used for anything except salad material and are almost never cooked. When these are listed, the amount per serving is given as unlimited and it is assumed that they are not cooked.

When the asterisk-marked vegetables are uncooked or lightly steamed they are considered as free foods, a category that has the color code of blue. See the next chapter for a fuller explanation. These low-density free foods give the person on a calorie-restricted diet an opportunity to feel "full" and not as "deprived" as he or she might be otherwise. The bonus in extra dietary fiber can help insure bowel regularity, not to mention the other real and theoretical benefits of the extra fiber, vitamins, and minerals from these foods.

43

This booklet will be used in the United Kingdom, so their vegetable terms will be used as well as those names used in this country.

FOOD NAME	AMOUNT PER SERVING FULLY COOKED
Alfalfa sprouts*	Unlimited
Artichoke, French or globe*	¹/₂ cup or ¹/₂ medium
Artichoke, Jerusalem*	¹/₂ cup
Asparagus* (A/C)	¹/₂ cup
Aubergine (Eggplant)	¹/₂ cup
Avocado — See Fat Portion List.	
Bamboo shoots or sprouts*	³/₄ cup
Beans — See Bread-Starch List.	
Bean sprouts*	¹/₂ cup
Beets (Beetroots)	¹/₂ cup
Beet greens*	¹/₂ cup (not usually steamed)
Bokchoy (Chinese cabbage) (A/C)	¹/₂ cup
Broccoli* (A/C)	¹/₂ cup
Brussels sprouts* (C)	¹/₂ cup
Cabbage* all types (C)	¹/₂ cup
Carrots (A)	¹/₂ cup
Cauliflower* (C)	¹/₂ cup
Celeriac* (root celery)	1 cup (high in sodium)
Celery*	1 cup (high in sodium)
Chard*	Unlimited
Chicory* (A)	Unlimited
Chilies*	Unlimited
Chinese leaves* (A/C)	¹/₂ cup
Chives* (A/C)	Unlimited
Cilantro or Coriander*	Unlimited
Collard greens or tops*(C)	¹/₂ cup
Corn — See Bread-Starch List.	
Courgettes (Zucchini)* (A/C)	¹/₂ cup
Cress*	Unlimited
Cucumber*	Unlimited
Dandelion greens or tops*	Unlimited
Eggplant	¹/₂ cup
Endive*	Unlimited

Escarole* (A)	Unlimited
Fennel* (A)	Unlimited
Garlic	Use in reasonable amounts
Green beans	¹/₂ cup
Green onion tops*	Unlimited
Green peas (Petits Pois)	¹/₂ cup
Green peppers, pimientos* (C)	¹/₂ cup
Kale* (A/C)	¹/₂ cup
Kohlrabi, Turnip cabbage (C)	¹/₂ cup
Laverbread	¹/₂ cup
Leeks (C)	¹/₂ cup
Lettuce, all kinds	Unlimited
Mangetout*	¹/₂ cup
Marrow* (A/C)	¹/₂ cup
Mint*	Unlimited
Mushrooms*	(Not usually ¹/₂ cup steamed)
Mustard greens or tops* (C)	¹/₂ cup
Okra, Ladies Fingers*	¹/₂ cup
Onions	¹/₂ cup
Parsley* (A/C)	Unlimited
Peas, shelled — See Bread-Starch List.	
Pea pods, Chinese	¹/₂ cup
Peas, English or green	¹/₂ cup
Pimentos*	¹/₂ cup
Poke*	Unlimited
Pumpkin (A)	¹/₂ cup
Radishes*	Unlimited
Red peppers* (C)	¹/₂ cup
Rhubarb*	¹/₂ cup
Romaine lettuce*	Unlimited
Rutabaga	¹/₂ cup
Salsify*	Unlimited
Sauerkraut	¹/₂ cup (high in sodium)
Seakale*	Unlimited
Shallots	¹/₂ cup
Spinach* (A/C)	¹/₂ cup
Spring greens* (A/C)	¹/₂ cup
Spring onions*	Unlimited

Squash, summer* (A/C)	¹/₂ cup
Squash, crookneck* (A/C)	¹/₂ cup
String beans	¹/₂ cup
Tomato, fresh (A/C)	1 large
Tomato/Vegetable juice	¹/₂ cup
	(Usually high in sodium)
Turnips	¹/₂ cup
Turnip greens (A/C)	¹/₂ cup
Water chestnuts	4 medium
Watercress* (A)	Unlimited
Waxbeans and other pod beans	¹/₂ cup
Zucchini squash* (A/C)	¹/₂ cup

Approved ways of cooking these vegetables, when they are to be fully cooked, include boiling, baking, steaming for more than five minutes, stewing, braising, and grilling without battering or the use of extra fats or oils.

For certain of the vegetables with a lower carbohydrate content, there may be some confusion in the quantities permitted per serving. These are, for the most part, the ones that have very little carbohydrate when uncooked or lightly steamed. Those with an asterisk (*) have far less available carbohydrate, even when cooked, than those with no marking. In previous exchange diets, a portion of these so-called "Group A" vegetables consisted of a full cup instead of a half-cup as noted above. We will go along with the new quantities since you can still get a respectable amount of these lower carbohydrate vegetables in the raw or lightly steamed states.

The Bread-Starch Food Group

These foods are either from grains, other seeds, or roots of plants. They are not all bread-like in appearance, but for our purposes they are essentially identical in nutritional composition to bread. Each portion contains about 80 calories, the equivalent of one slice of Malsovit bread, or 1¹/₂ Malsovit Mealwafers. Malsovit products should not be confused with so-called "low-calorie breads." Malsovit is a substantial, "stick to the ribs" bread with more than ample nutrients and fiber in contrast to the usual pale and empty calories of regular white bread. Where there are added fat calories to be accounted for, this is listed in the right-hand column. When it says "Omit ½ fat," this means that we have to account for an extra half-portion of fat, subtracting this from our daily allowance. On 1,000 and 1,200 calorie diets there are no fats or ways of earning fat bonuses by using a less fatty milk product. Therefore, those with these added fat calories cannot be used on those diets. Most people on maintenance will be on at least 1,500 calories a day, but the other charts are there if needed.

When it says "Omit ½ fruit," omit a half-portion of fruit from the daily allowance for each bread portion with that notation.

The bread portion group is represented by brown in my system of tracking food portions. Each brown item represents one portion from this group.

Breads and Baked Goods

TYPE OF PRODUCT	AMOUNT PER PORTION & TYPE	EXTRA PORTION
Bagel	½ bagel	
Biscuits from mix	1 biscuit	Omit ½ fat
Biscuit, buttermilk	1 biscuit	Omit ½ fat
Biscuit, flaky	1 biscuit	Omit 1 fat
Bread, Hollywood	1 slice	
Bread, rye	1 slice	
Bread, white or French	1 slice	
Bread, whole wheat	1 slice	
Breadsticks, crisp	4"x½" 2 sticks	(²/₃ oz.)
Bun, Hamburger/ Frankfurter	½ bun	(1 oz.)
Cornbread square	1 piece, 1½"	Omit 1 fat
Croutons, plain	½ cup	
English muffin	½ muffin	
Malsovit bread	1 slice	
Malsovit Mealwafer	1½ wafers	
Matzo cracker	1 cracker, 6" square	
Melba toast	5 pieces	

Muffin, bran, homemade	1 2" muffin	Omit 1 fat
Muffin, corn, homemade	1 2" muffin	Omit 1 fat
Pancakes from mix	2 pancakes, 3" diam.	
Pita bread	1/2 of 6" pocket	
Popover from mix	1/2 popover	Omit 1/2 fat
Raisin bread, unfrosted	1 slice	
Rice cakes	2 cakes	
Roll, brown & serve	1 roll	Omit 1/2 fat
Roll, butterflake	1 roll	Omit 1/2 fat
Roll, crescent	1 roll	Omit 1 fat
Roll, croissant, Sara Lee	1 roll	Omit 1 fat
Roll, all others	1 roll 2" diam.	
Rusks	2 rusks	
Spoon bread	2 oz. (1/4 cup)	Omit 1 fat
Taco/Tostada shell	2 shells	Omit 1 fat
Tortilla	1 tortilla, 6" diam.	
Waffle	1 waffle, 4" square	

Cereals and Pasta

TYPE OF PRODUCT	AMOUNT PER PORTION & TYPE	EXTRA PORTION
All Bran	1/3 cup	
Alpha Bits	3/4 cup	
Apple Jacks	1 cup	Omit 1 fruit
Bran, 100%	1/2 cup	
Bran Buds	1/3 cup	
Bran Chex	1/2 cup	
Bran Flakes, 40%	1/2 cup	
Buc Wheats	1/2 cup	
Bulgur (cooked)	1/2 cup	
Cap'n Crunch	3/4 cup	Omit 1/2 fat
Cheerios	3/4 cup	
Cocoa Krispies & Pebbles	3/4 cup	Omit 1 fruit
Cocoa Puffs	1 cup	Omit 1 fruit
Cooked cereals not listed	1/2 cup	
Corn bran	1/2 cup	
Corn Chex	1/2 cup	
Corn flakes	3/4 cup	

48

Corn grits, cooked	1/2 cup	
Corn meal, dry	2 1/2 tablespoons	
Corn Total	3/4 cup	
Count Chocula	1 cup	Omit 1 fruit
Cream of Rice, cooked	1/2 cup	
Cream of Wheat, cooked	1/2 cup	
Farina, cooked	1/2 cup	
Fortified oat flakes	1/2 cup	
Frankenberry	1 cup	Omit 1 fruit
Froot Loops	1 cup	Omit 1 fruit
Frosted Miniwheats	4 biscuits	Omit 1 fruit
Fruit & Fibre	2/3 cup	Omit 1/2 fruit
Grape Nuts	1/4 cup = 1 1/2 portions	
Grape Nuts Flakes	2/3 cup	
Grits, cooked	1/2 cup	
Heartland Natural Cereals	1/4 cup of any	Omit 1 fat
Honeycomb	2/3 cup	
Kix	1 cup	
Life, plain & cinnamon	2/3 cup	Omit 1 fruit
Lucky Charms	1 cup	Omit 1 fruit
Macaroni, cooked	1/2 cup	
Most	1/2 cup	
Noodles, cooked	1/2 cup	
Noodles, Chow Mein	1/4 cup	
Nutrigrain, all types	1/2 cup	
Oats, regular, cooked	1/2 cup	
Pasta, all types, cooked	1/2 cup	
Product 19	1/2 cup	
Puffed rice or wheat	1 1/2 cup	
Raisin bran	1/2 cup	
Rice Chex	3/4 cup	
Rice Krispies, plain	2/3 cup	
Roman Meal, cooked	1/2 cup	
Shredded Wheat	1 large biscuit or 1/2 cup	
Spaghetti, cooked, no sauce	1/3 cup	
Special K	1 1/3 cups	Omit 1 fruit

Sugar-coated cereals	Not recommended unless listed	
Team	²/₃ cup	
Total	²/₃ cup	
Trix	²/₃ cup	
Wheat Chex	¹/₂ cup	
Wheat & Raisin Chex	¹/₂ cup	Omit 1 fruit
Wheatena, cooked	¹/₂ cup	
Wheaties	²/₃ cup	

Starchy Vegetables and Legumes

TYPE OF PRODUCT	AMOUNT PER PORTION
Beans, dried, cooked	¹/₃ cup
Beans, baked without pork	¹/₄ cup
Corn, cooked	¹/₂ cup
Corn on cob	1 piece, 6″ long
Hominy, cooked	¹/₂ cup
Lentils, dried, cooked	¹/₃ cup
Lima beans, cooked	¹/₂ cup
Parsnips, cooked	1 small
Peas, dried, cooked	¹/₃ cup
Peas, green, cooked	¹/₂ cup
Plantain	¹/₂ cup
Potato, sweet/yam, cooked	¹/₃ cup
Potato, white, baked	1 small, 3 oz.
Potatoes, white, mashed	¹/₂ cup
Squash, winter, acorn	³/₄ cup
Squash, winter, butternut	³/₄ cup

Crackers and Snacks

TYPE OF PRODUCT	AMOUNT PER PORTION & TYPE	EXTRA PORTION
Animal crackers	8 crackers	
Graham crackers	3 crackers, 2¹/₂″ square	
Oyster crackers	24 crackers	
Popcorn, airpopped only	3 cups	
Pretzels	³/₄ ounces	
Ritz and similar crackers	5 crackers	Omit 1 fat

Rye Krisp	3 crackers
Saltines	6 small squares
Triscuits	4 crackers
Uneeda biscuits	4 biscuits

The Meat and Meat-Like Portion List

It is difficult for someone on a diet to learn what constitutes a meat-like food and how to calculate values of a meat portion. The foods listed here are in this group and are coded according to whether there is a low, medium, or high content of fat in each portion. Each portion has about seven grams of protein, but the fat content varies from three grams per low-fat portion, to five grams per medium-fat portion, all the way up to eight grams of fat in each of the high-fat portions. This gives each portion 55, 75, or 100 calories, depending on the amount of fat contained in the protein food.

The weights given are for lean cuts, with all fat, bones, and skin trimmed off prior to cooking. Four ounces of raw meat will usually weight three ounces when cooked. So that you can make accurate decisions as to fat content, I am marking the low-fat protein foods with two asterisks (**) and the moderate-fat ones with one asterisk (*). Those with a high fat content are not marked at all. It is better to limit your choices from this last group to no more than three times a week. If eggs are eaten and cholesterol is a problem, it is usually better to have no more than three a week.

During the weight reduction phase of your diet, limit the consumption of canned meats and fatty meat pies severely because of their extremely high fat content. Cheese and other fermented milk products are listed here because of their protein content. They are still a good source of calcium, but the fat content must be carefully considered in your selection of these foods.

Each quantity listed below is equal to one meat or meat-like portion. This is also equal to a meat exchange if you are referring to a diabetic food exchange list. All weights given are cooked weights, with the cooking done in the appropriate way, using or retaining minimal fat in the cooking process. One ounce is also equal to 28 grams of boneless, trimmed weight. Some foods are higher in sodium and are marked with a capital "S" to signify that fact.

FOOD NAME	AMOUNT PER PORTION
Abalone**	1¹/₃ oz.
Anchovies, canned, drained** S	1 oz. or 9 fillets
Bacon-Not counted as a meat— See Fat Portion List.	
Bass**	1¹/₂ oz.
Beef, good or choice, lean**	1 oz.
Flank, round, & sirloin**	1 oz.
Tenderloin**	1 oz.
Chipped beef **S	1 oz.
Beef, prime grades (ribs)	1 oz.
Beef, corned S	1 oz.
Beef, brisket, lean and fat*	1 oz.
Beef, forerib, lean*	1 oz.
Beef, ground, lean, drained*	1 oz.
Beef liver, kidney, tongue	1 oz.
Beef heart, brains	1 oz.
Beef, lean rump steak, grilled*	1 oz.
Beef, roasts and steaks*	1 oz.
Beef meatloaf*	1 oz.
Canadian bacon	1 slice ¹/₄″ thick x 3″ diameter
Cheese, American S	1 oz.
Cheese, blue, Monterey, Swiss S	1 oz.
Cheese, cheddar S	1 oz.
Cheese, cottage, low-fat**	¹/₄ cup
Cheese, cottage, 4% milkfat	¹/₄ cup
Cheese, Edam, Gruyere*	1 oz.
Cheese, Parmesan, grated	2 tablespoons
Cheese, diet, *S	1 oz. of less than 55 cal/oz. cheese
Cheese, farmer's, hoop, or pot**	¹/₄ cup
Cheese, Mozzarella*	1 oz.
Cheese, ricotta*	¹/₄ cup
Cheese from Soya Milk*S	1 oz.
Chicken, light or dark meat**	1 oz. without skin
Chicken with skin*	1 oz.

Chicken livers, heart, or gizzard	1 oz.
Clams, raw**S	2 oz.
Cod**	1 oz.
Cold cuts, regular type	1 slice, $^1/_8''$ thick x 4 $^1/_2''$ diameter
Cold cuts, 86% fat-free S	1 oz. or 1 slice
Cold cuts, 95% fat-free S	1 oz. or 1 slice
Cornish hen, without skin**	1 oz.
Crabmeat, canned or fresh**S	2 oz. steamed
Duck, wild, without skin**	1 oz.
Duck, domestic, without skin*	1 oz.
Eggs, cooked any way without fat*	1 egg
Egg whites**	3 whites (from 3 eggs)
Egg substitutes,	
Egg substitutes 56-80 cal/oz.	$^1/_4$ cup
Fish, all types not specified*	1 oz. not fried or breaded
Fish, fried	1 oz.
Flounder**	1 oz.
Frankfurter, beef and/or pork S	1 (10/lb.) give up 1 fat per portion
Frankfurter, chicken or turkey S	1 (10/lb.)
Goose, without skin, wild**	1 oz.
Goose, domestic, without skin*	1 oz.
Haddock or Halibut**	1 oz.
Ham, fresh, lean*	1 oz.
Ham, canned, cured, or boiled**S	1 oz.
Herring, uncreamed or smoked**S	1 oz.
Knockwurst, smoked S	1 oz.
Lamb, lean, chop or roast**	1 oz.
Lamb patties (ground lamb)	1 oz.
Lobster, fresh or canned**	1 oz.
Luncheon meat (bologna, salami) S	1 oz. or 1 slice
Oysters	6 medium
Peanut butter	1 tablespoon
Pheasant, wild	1 oz.
Pork, lean chops or cutlets*	1 oz.

Pork, loin roast & Boston butt*	**1 oz.**
Pork sausage S	**1 patty, $^1/_4''$ thick x 3 $^1/_2''$ diameter**
Pork spareribs 1 oz.	
Rabbit	**1 oz.**
SalmonS**	**1 oz. fresh, or 1$^1/_2$ oz canned**
Sardines, well-drained of oil*	**2 medium**
Sausage, Polish or Italian S	**1 oz.**
ScallopsS**	**3 medium or 1$^1/_2$ oz.**
Shrimp, fresh or cannedS**	**2 oz. or 6 shrimp**
Soy beans, cooked	**$^1/_4$ cup**
Squirrel**	**1 oz.**
Tofu*	**1 portion 2$^1/_2''$ x 2 $^3/_4''$ x 1''**
Turkey, light or dark meat**	**1 oz.**
Tuna, water packedS**	**$^1/_4$ cup**
Veal, lean, loin cut, chops**	**1 oz.**
Veal cutlet, ground or cubed*	**1 oz. unbreaded**
Venison	**1 oz.**

Free Foods

This category of food is represented by the color blue. You really do not have to keep track of free foods, except where there is an amount following the name of the product. Certain of the vegetable foods are marked as being permitted in unlimited amounts. This would be whether the vegetable were raw or lightly steamed as described. These vegetables are not listed here but are still considered in this category.

FOOD NAME

Bouillon or broth, without fat (Better as low-sodium)
Candy, hard, sugar-free (Two small pieces)
Carbonated drinks, sugar-free
Catsup, non-diet (One teaspoon daily)
Catsup, diet or imitation (Two teaspoons daily)
Chili sauce, diet, Featherweight or similar brand (Two teaspoons daily)
Cocoa powder, unsweetened (One tablespoon)
Coffee

Cranberries, unsweetened or with artificial sweeteners ($^1/_2$ cup)
Drink mixes, sugar-free (Crystal Light, Kool-Aid)
Extract of almond, lemon, chocolate, or vanilla (Total of two tablespoons daily
Gelatin, unflavored
Gelatin, sugar-free
Gum, sugar-free (Two pieces)
Hot sauce (Two teaspoons daily)
Horseradish, plain, not the creamy mixtures
Jam or jelly, sugar-free (Two teaspoons)
Mustard
Pancake syrup, sugar-free (Two tablespoons)
Pickles, dill, unsweetened
Rhubarb, unsweetened ($^1/_2$ cup)
Salad dressing, low-calorie (Maximum of 25 calories a day)
Taco sauce (Two tablespoons)
Tea
Tonic water, sugar-free
Vinegar

These free foods are useful in filling out your daily intake of food and making things more interesting and tasty.

Spices Used in Cooking

The following spices are also permitted in reasonable amounts with the foods listed:

Artichokes — bay leaves, marjoram, thyme.

Asparagus — caraway seed, mustard, nutmeg, sesame seed, tarragon.

Beans, green — basil, bay leaves, cloves, curry, dill, marjoram, mustard, nutmeg, oregano, savory, sesame seeds, tarragon, thyme.

Beans, lima — celery seed, chili powder, curry, oregano, sage.

Beets — allspice, bay leaves, caraway seeds, cloves, ginger.

Broccoli — caraway seed, marjoram, mustard, oregano, tarragon.

Brussels sprouts — caraway seed, mustard, nutmeg, sage.

Cabbage — allspice, basil, caraway seed, celery seed, cumin, curry powder, dill, fennel, mustard, nutmeg, oregano, savory, tarragon.

Carrots — allspice, bay leaves, caraway seed, celery seed, chives, cinnamon, cloves, curry, dill, ginger, mace, marjoram, mint, nutmeg, savory, tarragon, thyme.

Cauliflower — caraway seed, cayenne, celery seed, curry, dill, marjoram, mustard, nutmeg, oregano, paprika, rosemary, savory, tarragon.

Corn — cayenne, celery seed, chili powder, chives, curry, paprika.

Eggplant — allspice, basil, bay leaves, chili powder, marjoram, sage, thyme.

Mushrooms — marjoram, rosemary, tarragon, thyme.

Onions — basil, bay leaves, caraway seed, chili powder, curry, ginger, mustard, nutmeg, oregano, paprika, sage, thyme.

Peas — basil, chili powder, dill, marjoram, mint, mustard, oregano, poppy seed, rosemary, sage.

Potatoes, Sweet — allspice, cardamon, cinnamon, cloves, ginger, nutmeg, poppy seed.

Potatoes, white — basil, bay leaves, caraway seed, celery seed, chives, dill, fennel, mace, mustard, oregano, paprika, rosemary, savory, sesame seed, thyme.

Spinach — allspice, basil, cinnamon, dill, mace, marjoram, nutmeg, oregano, rosemary, sesame seed.

Summer Squash — basil, bay leaves, cardomon, mace, marjoram, mustard, rosemary.

Winter Squash — allspice, basil, cardamon, cinnamon, cloves, ginger, marjoram, nutmeg, paprika.

Tomatoes — basil, bay leaves, caraway seed, celery seed, chili powder, cloves, curry, dill, garlic, marjoram, oregano, rosemary, sage, savory, sesame seed, thyme.

Turnips — allspice, caraway seed, celery seed, dill, oregano.

PORTION LISTS FOR CALORIE-CONTROLLED MEAL PLANNING

Calories per day	Food	Portions	Bkfast	Lunch	Dinner	Total Cal.
1,000	Milk*	1	0	1	2	180
	Vegetable	0	0	1	1	25
	Meat (mod-fat)	1	2	2	5	375
	Fruit	1	1	1	3	180
	Bread-Starch	1	1	1	3	240
	Fat	0	0	0	0	---
1,200 (1,195)	Milk*	1	0	1	2	180
	Vegetable	0	1	1	2	50
	Meat (mod-fat)	1	2	2	5	375
	Fruit	1	1	1	3	180
	Bread-Starch	1	2	1	4	320
	Fat	1	0	1	2	90
1,400 (1,415)	Milk	1	0	1	2	300
	Vegetable	0	1	2	3	75
	Meat	1	2	3	6	450
	Fruit	1	1	1	3	180
	Bread-Starch	1	2	1	4	320
	Fat	1	0	1	2	90
1,500 (1,495)	Milk	1	0	1	2	300
	Vegetable	0	1	2	3	75
	Meat	1	2	3	6	450
	Fruit	1	1	1	3	180
	Bread-Starch	2	2	1	5	400
	Fat	1	0	1	2	90
1,600 (1,620)	Milk	1	0	1	2	300
	Vegetable	0	1	2	3	75
	Meat	1	2	3	6	450
	Fruit	1	1	1	3	180
	Bread-Starch	2	2	2	6	480
	Fat	1	1	1	3	135
1,800	Milk	1	0	1	2	300
	Vegetable	0	2	2	4	100
	Meat	2	2	3	7	525
	Fruit	1	1	1	3	180
	Bread-Starch	2	3	2	7	560
	Fat	1	1	1	3	135

57

PORTION LISTS FOR CALORIE-CONTROLLED MEAL PLANNING

Calories per day	Food	Portions	Bkfast	Lunch	Dinner Cal.	Total
2,000 (2015)	Milk	1	0	1	2	300
	Vegetable	0	2	2	4	100
	Meat (mod-fat)	2	3	3	8	600
	Fruit	1	1	2	4	240
	Bread-Starch	2	3	3	8	640
	Fat	1	1	1	3	135
2,200 (2215)	Milk	1	0	1	2	300
	Vegetable	0	2	2	4	100
	Meat (mod-fat)	2	3	4	9	675
	Fruit	1	1	2	4	240
	Bread-Starch	3	3	3	9	720
	Fat	1	2	1	4	180
2,400 (2405)	Milk	1	1	1	3	450
	Vegetable	0	2	2	4	100
	Meat (mod-fat)	2	3	4	9	675
	Fruit	1	2	1	4	240
	Bread-Starch	3	3	3 $1/2$	9 $1/2$	760
	Fat	1	2	1	4	180
2,600	Milk	1	1	1	3	450
	Vegetable	0	2	2	4	100
	Meat (mod-fat)	3	3	4	10	750
	Fruit	1	2	1	4	240
	Bread-Starch	3	4	4	11	880
	Fat	1	2	1	4	180
2,800 (2815)	Milk	1	1	1	3	450
	Vegetable	0	2	2	4	100
	Meat (mod-fat)	3	4	4	11	825
	Fruit	2	2	1	5	300
	Bread-Starch	4	4	4	12	960
	Fat	1	2	1	4	180
3,000 (2970)	Milk	1	1	1	3	450
	Vegetable	0	2	2	4	100
	Meat (mod-fat)	4	4	4	12	900
	Fruit	2	2	1	5	300
	Bread-Starch	4	5	4	13	1040
	Fat	1	2	1	4	180

When no milk is allowed, substitute one moderate-fat meat and one fruit for each portion of regular milk. In the 1,000 and 1,200 calorie diets, there are no fat bonuses and the milk products used are always of the very low-fat type. On diets above 1,200 calories, the milk is whole milk and the fat portion bonuses apply when a milk product of lower fat content is used.

It is expected that a variety of meats will be used with an average calorie content of about 75 calories for each portion. All portions on this and the preceding page may be moved to any part of the day, just as long as all of the portions of that category of food are consumed before the end of the day.

The calorie charts on the preceding pages will be used by you and your doctor to determine how much food you eat each day, and in what proportions you have this food. You may use your bonus system on diets that exceed 1,200 calories and get extra fat portions when lower fat milk items are used. The guidelines for using lower fat meats are still in effect unless you are told otherwise.

A lot of different foods are included here but not nearly so many as you will find at your supermarket. A good number of those foods are combination foods, with several different food groups represented in their makeup. In order to give the dieter something to work with, I am including a substantial number of commercial foods with their exchange information supplied. No endorsement of any of these foods is implied. They are included for the convenience of the people using this book. The lists of these commercial foods are to be found in Chapter 13.

Alcoholic beverage values are included, but these beverages should generally only be used after the desired weight is reached. Should you then choose to use them, you must give up the listed amounts of food portions for that day that correspond to a drink. An example would be one ounce of 97 proof spirits in a noncaloric mixer. This amount of alcohol contains the calories and is burned like two fat portions (90 calories). If you and your doctor decide you can have a drink, you must give up those two fat portions for that day.

After a while you can use the information on an individual food package for the nutritional content and start making your own decisions about mixed food selections. Until then, use the tables given at the end of this book. Don't hesitate to ask your physician or his staff, including a dietician referred by him or her, if there are questions.

It is still a good idea to use the Malsovit high-fiber bread or the Malsovit Mealwafers during maintenance. About five slices of Malsovit bread (three in the morning and two for lunch), or six of the Malsovit Mealwafers (or a combination), are suggested for each day. Be selective in the type of starch you consume and make sure that there is adequate fiber and protein in each selection.

CHAPTER FOUR

FOOD MEASUREMENT AND PREPARATION WITH SELECTED RECIPES

It is important to get food quantities correct, whether the amount per portion is given in fluid ounces, ounces of weight, dimensions in inches, or other units. Many people are still unsure about what constitutes a cup, or an ounce, relying on their own unsure judgement to help with the measurement. It is always better to use proper measurement technique, at least in the initial stages of the program.

Once you become proficient in measurement and estimation of portion size, it will not be as necessary for you to do these measurements every time. The basic items needed, as mentioned earlier, include several measuring cups, a set of plastic or metal teaspoon to tablespoon measuring sets, a ruler, and a scale, preferably with a dish attachment for convenience.

Using water for fluid measurement practice and uncooked rice or beans for checking on how the quantities of one cup, one-half cup, etc., look on a plate or in a glass is helpful. For your information I have given some common equivalent units of measurement below.

One teaspoon (t.) equals about ¹/₆ fluid ounce.
Three t. equals one tablespoon (T.).
Two T. equals one fluid ounce.
Eight fluid ounces equals one cup.
Four fluid ounces equals ¹/₂ cup.
Sixteen ounces of weight equals one pound.
One kilogram equals about 2.2 pounds.
One ounce of weight equals about 28.5 grams.
100 grams is slightly over three ounces.
100 milliliters is slightly over three fluid ounces.
One liter is slightly over one quart.

It is better if you use your own glasses, cups, plates and bowls when you are practicing your measurement of quantities. This makes it a lot easier to do estimates of portion amounts later. When using salad dressings, be sure and measure carefully. The soup ladles used in some restaurants to measure their 100 calories/ounce dressing or their 60 calories/ounce "diet dressing" are too generous. It is possible to be careless and put 500 or more calories per ladle of dressing on your salad.

Be consistent in your measurements and you should do quite well. On the next two pages are some drawings of five different portions of meat or poultry, provided by Carnrick Labs, Inc. and used with their permission. These drawings came from U.S. Government sources originally and are quite accurate.

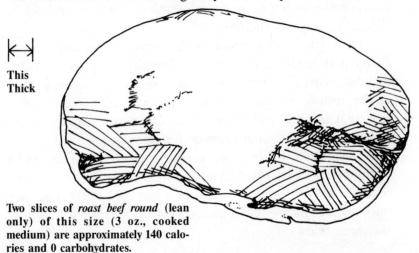

This Thick

Two slices of *roast beef round* (lean only) of this size (3 oz., cooked medium) are approximately 140 calories and 0 carbohydrates.

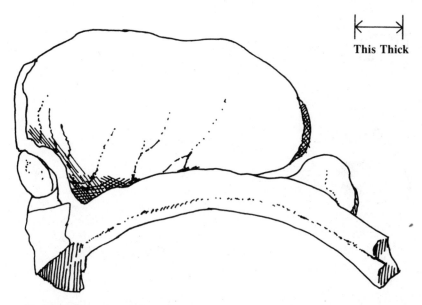

This Thick

Two *pork chops* (lean only) of this size (3 oz., cooked medium) are approximately 230 calories and 0 carbohydrates.

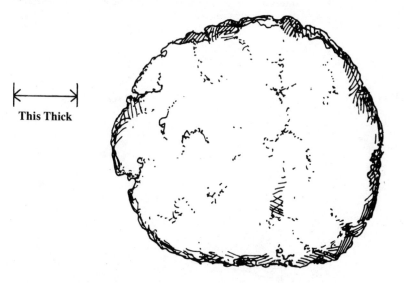

This Thick

One *hamburger* (lean only) of this size (3 oz., cooked medium) is approximately 185 calories and 0 carbohydrates.

This Thick

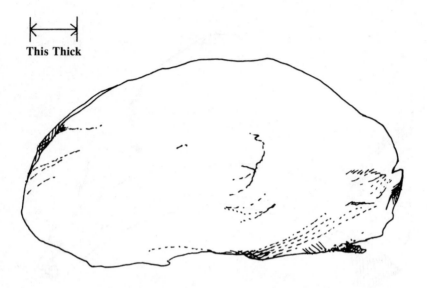

Two slices of this size (3 oz., cooked) of the light meat of a *roast turkey* are approximately 150 calories and 0 carbohydrates. Two slices of this size (3 oz. cooked) of the dark meat of a *roast turkey* are approximately 175 calories and 0 carbohydrates.

This Thick

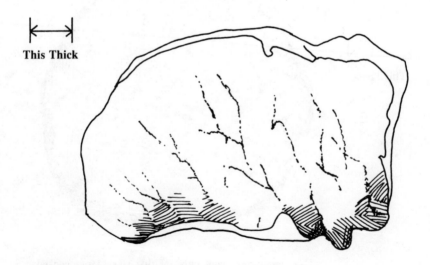

One *veal cutlet* (trimmed) of this size (3 oz., cooked medium) is approximately 185 calories and 0 carbohydrates.

FOOD PREPARATION

The biggest enemy of a dieter or slimmer is excess fat in the diet. Fat is the most concentrated of all nutrients and must be dealt with by changing the way foods are cooked.

Many of the patients and friends I have observed still use too much butter, lard, cream, margarine, cream cheese, and oils in their cooking. Instead of using rich, creamy sauces and gravies, I have encouraged them to utilize the natural juices of the foods and to avoid smothering the actual flavors of the foods in too many spices and condiments.

Preparation of beef, chicken, and fish stocks for soups is a relatively simple procedure. The majority of the fats present are removed by the process of refrigerating the stock and getting rid of the upper layer of fat after the liquid has cooked sufficiently for the fats to solidify. These stocks are then available for the preparation of delicious soups, "dieter's gravies," and other flavor enhancers that increase the taste pleasure of a meal without increasing the calories very much. Jeanne Jones, noted author, gourmet cook, and nutritionist, has a number of excellent low-fat and low-calorie cookbooks on the market. I would suggest you check your local book store for some of her books.

Just because we limit fat doesn't mean to say that the person who reaches his or her goal cannot indulge the palate, usually with no penalty in weight gain. The cooking techniques mentioned below are by no means the only way to prepare food but are given as a basic guide for the busy slimmer.

BOILING

It is usually better to boil vegetables in an open pan with lots of water. Bring the water to a boil, usually with a minimum amount of salt added, and carefully place the vegetables into the water. Bring to a boil and let the cover stay off the saucepan. Cook the recommended amount of time, followed by draining in a colander. Serve as soon as possible.

There are cooks who say that a minimum amount of water in a covered pan does better, but I usually utilize the Cordon Bleu method, with an open pan and lots of boiling water.

Parboiling is a variant of boiling. Vegetables that are dense, usually root vegetables, are partially cooked by boiling and then are fried without grease or fats to complete the cooking process. Parboiling is fine, provided the frying is done on Teflon or a non-stick cooking surface of some other type, including a regular pan sprayed with PAM. I personally prefer Pommes Frites a la Cooper, for example, as a relatively fat-free parboiled dish.

I take three or four medium-sized potatoes and boil in lightly-salted water for about nine or ten minutes. The excess water is drained off and the potatoes are immediately cut into ¼ inch slices. They are lightly dusted with butter salt, Molly McButter, or other condiments to taste, and then are browned on a non-stick pan surface. The resulting chips or pommes frites are crisp and tasty, but without any fat added, as would be the case in deep frying. On the slimming portion of the diet, it is better to use little or no salt. On the maintenance portion, you may indulge in salt if you have no fluid retention problems.

Neither mushrooms nor tomatoes should be boiled or parboiled, at least for use as a vegetable accompaniment to an entree. In soups or sauces this does not apply.

Most meats, fish, seafood, and poultry can be boiled or parboiled. The rich stocks and juices from this process can be used as flavor enhancers once the fat has been removed.

STEAMING

Certain vegetables, including beets, kohlrabi, yams, sweet potatoes, and tomatoes, should not be steamed. The remainder of those listed in this booklet are usually suitable for full cooking by steaming, or partial cooking for five minutes or less on a stovetop or counter steamer. You don't usually steam "greens" like collards or turnip greens, but some people do.

Steaming for five minutes or less will preserve the vitamins and minerals and will not break down the cellulose structure of a vegetable so that it has usable calories for the slimmer to absorb. If a vegetable is a free-use one (blue category), with unlimited amounts permitted if not fully cooked, it must be cooked no longer than the five minutes allotted in the steamer.

Almost any meat, poultry, or fish dish can be prepared by steaming. The trick is to steam it long enough, particularly the poultry, to properly cook it. Any of several good cookbooks have steaming times for various foods.

FRYING

Remember that fat is a slimmer's enemy. Use about a tenth of what you think you need when you measure out cooking oils or fats. If possible, use none at all! Teflon and non-stick pan sprays are excellent aids that permit you to cook without burning foods and without extra and unwanted calories. Instead of deep-frying, try parboiling and grilling instead.

Wok cooking is an acceptable variant if properly used. A carbon steel wok with a minimum amount of oil at the bottom is often useful. Stir frying is an art and takes practice but produces a minimum amount of extra fat calories to burden the slimmer. Read directions carefully before using one of these utensils.

BAKING

This is another one of my favorite methods of cooking foods. Fruits and vegetables retain their flavor but get very few fat calories in this type of cooking. Meats and other protein foods, if allowed to lose their fatty juices into a pan underneath the baking rack, will have a much lower fat content per ounce than otherwise. The provision for a dripping space between the bottom edge of the cooking meat and the drip pan will eliminate the possibility that a lot of unwanted fat will be retained in the joint of beef or other meat.

COOKING WITH WINE

There is nothing wrong with using wine as a flavor enhancer, provided that the alcohol can evaporate during the cooking process. Avoid sauces that are swimming in wine and that still have their alcohol content unaltered.

GRILLING

I use either a charcoal or a Jennair grill when I cook certain cuts of meat, poultry, and fish. In the United States we use a type of wood called mesquite, which lends a different flavor to the cooked meats. The resulting meat dishes produced by this open method of grilling are quite delicious and have a far lower fat content because of the loss of fatty drippings that fall into the coals or the fire. The fatty drippings are consumed by the hot coals and the smoke comes back up to permeate the meat, producing another unique flavor.

Vegetables to be grilled over coals should be wrapped with foil or other protective coatings (corn husks, etc.). Potatoes and sweet corn are excellent for grilling, but you might try your own favorites to see how they do.

In summary, for all these methods of cooking, use as little fat as possible and try to preserve the natural flavors of the foods, rather than trying to smother them with fatty and high-calorie sauces and gravies.

RECIPES FOR SLIMMERS AND DIETERS

Most of these can be used in the fat-losing stage of the diet, as well as the maintenance period. Where they are not suitable for the Dutch Diet, there is a notation to that effect.

Paddington's Quiche

Take eight one-ounce slices of mozzarella cheese, six beaten eggs, four fluid ounces unsweetened low-fat yogurt, $1/2$ teaspoon salt. Also take either 12 ounces boiled shrimp or prawns, or ten ounces chopped lean ham, or ten ounces ground lean beef. Any of these three selections should be pre-cooked, drained of all excess grease, blotted with a paper towel, and finely chopped into small fragments.

Preheat oven to 375 degrees. Line a round pie or quiche pan evenly with the eight slices of mozzarella cheese to make the "crust" for the quiche. Take the six beaten eggs and combine in a bowl with yogurt and salt. Mix well and pour into pan. Sprinkle either the shrimp, ham, or beef evenly into mixture in pan. Garnish with a small amount of chopped green peppers, celery, or raw mushrooms if desired. Bake for 25 minutes in preheated oven. Remove from heat and let stand for at least ten minutes before serving. Cut into eight wedges. Each wedge contains three high-fat meat portions. Use sparingly, and no more than twice a week.

Tuna (or Salmon) Crispies

Take six ounces water-packed tuna or salmon. Drain well. Mix in $1/4$ cup finely chopped celery, one beaten egg, 2 teaspoons Worchestershire sauce, and salt and pepper to taste. After mixture is completely blended together, shape into two equal patties. Fry on non-stick surface without grease or oil until brown on both sides. Each crispie contains two low-fat meat portions. This recipe is one that Jeanne Jones and I have had a lot of laughs about. She thinks that the usual product of this recipe resembles a couple of hockey pucks, but I found them quite delicious. Try it and see what you think.

Diet Berry Pie Treat

This recipe was given to me by a patient. I don't know the source, but I am pleased with its taste. Each portion of pie equals one fruit portion.

Take one envelope unflavored gelatin, $1/4$ teaspoon cinnamon, $1/2$ teaspoon butter flavoring, one tablespoon lemon juice, four ounces diet Shasta Grape or some other diet grape soda, 2 packs Sweet'n Low, and three cups frozen, whole, unsweetened berries (any kind). Divide the berries into a one-cup and a two-cup portion.

Soften gelatin in four ounces water. Crush one cup of berries on top of double boiler and cook with diet grape soda. Add lemon juice, butter flavoring, cinnamon, and artificial sweetener. Equal is not used because heat destroys it during cooking. Add softened gelatin and cook for five more minutes. Cool ten minutes, then fold in remaining two cups of whole berries. Pour into chilled pie pan and place in refrigerator for three hours. Serve chilled. Cut pie into six pieces. Each piece equals 60 calories, or one fruit portion.

Pasta Salad

Take three different shapes of soft cooked pasta (not al dente). The rotini, wheels, and macaroni elbows are good in this type of dish. Add one cup of each type of cooked pasta to a large bowl. Pasta should be cool at time of mixing. Chop up three large stalks of broccoli so that no piece is larger than will fit in a teaspoon without overlapping. Chop up one large carrot into coin-shaped slices. Add two ounces of diet Italian dressing to the bowl after the chopped vegetables. Toss and mix thoroughly. Divide the mixture into three salad bowls. Sprinkle ½ teaspoon grated Parmesan cheese over the salad. Each serving is equal to two bread-starch portions.

This recipe is not for use during the active phase of the Dutch Diet, but it is fine for maintenance.

A Low-Calorie Bran Muffin Recipe

This is another recipe that was contributed by a patient. Take three tablespoons nonfat dry milk solids, three tablespoons water, two envelopes Sweet'n Low, ¾ cored apple, ¼ teaspoon vanilla extract, four drops almond extract, a pinch of cinnamon, a pinch of nutmeg, and five to six tablespoons unprocessed wheat or oat bran. Put all ingredients except bran into a blender. Blend at medium speed until apple is chunky. Pour into a bowl and add bran. Whip batter with spoon and mix well. Divide batter among four cupcake holders and bake at 350 degrees for 35 minutes. Yield is four muffins. Four muffins equal a total of one low-fat milk portion and one fruit portion. These muffins are more for the maintenance program but could be used once a week as a snack choice to replace a milk-fruit snack.

Diet Gazpacho

Take one whole onion, one large green pepper, two whole tomatoes (fresh is preferred), two medium cucumbers (remove all seeds from cucumbers and pepper), one tablespoon vegetable oil, a pinch of cumin spice, a level teaspoon of fructose (optional), one tablespoon cider vinegar, one teaspoon lemon juice. Chop onion, pepper, and cucumbers in food processor. Add tomatoes, one at a time, and continue processing until liquid. Add balance of ingredients and totally liquefy. Strain to remove large particles. Refrigerate and serve cold.

Au Gratin Eggplant Soup

Take a three-quart soup pot or pan. Spray Pam or other non-stick spray on pot or pan. Add one large onion and two celery stalks that have been finely chopped in a food processor or on a cutting board. Allow the onion and celery to cook slowly until soft. Stir in two cloves of garlic, finely chopped, and cook for two more minutes. Stir in two medium-sized eggplants (aubergines), finely chopped, along with 1/2 teaspoon each of dried thyme and ground coriander seed. Sauté for three minutes more on low heat, then add a medium-sized red pepper that has been finely diced. Add one quart of low-sodium beef broth, chicken broth, or other low-calorie soup that has no more than 80 to 90 calories per 15-ounce can. Low-sodium stock may be used as well. Bring the mixture to a boil, cover, and let simmer for at least 30 minutes.

Add two tablespoons chopped coriander leaves. Place soup in Pyrex or similar bowl, place a tomato slice on top of each soup serving. Sprinkle with liberal amounts of grated Swiss cheese, and lightly broil until cheese has melted. Serve at once. Limit this soup to one serving of six to eight ounces per day.

Mock Spaghetti Sauce

Take one cup vinegar, 1/2 cup catsup, one clove garlic, two tablespoons Worchestershire sauce, one teaspoon liquid non-caloric sweetener with saccharin, one teaspoon dry mustard, 1/2 teaspoon Tabasco sauce, 1 teaspoon salt.

Mix together all ingredients and simmer ten minutes in a saucepan. Each tablespoon contains ten calories. You may use up to four tablespoons (two ounces) daily on pasta. Any unused portion can be stored in a closed container in your refrigerator and warmed for use as needed. Both this and the next sauce are only used during maintenance.

Mock Spaghetti Sauce with Meat

Make up the above mixture and pour two ounces into a measuring cup. Take three ounces, raw weight, of *very* lean ground chuck. Brown on a non-stick surface, stirring frequently. Make sure meat is fully cooked and then drain off excess grease. Pour in two ounces of mock sauce and allow to simmer for five minutes over very low heat. Add to pasta and enjoy! Equals one fruit portion and three meat portions, plus the bread-starch portions represented by the pasta.

Both sauce recipes are courtesy of Dr. Dick Brennan of Houston.

Dr. Cooper's Super Soup

Take two green peppers, several whole tomatoes, five large onions, one large head of cabbage, and one large celery bunch. Seasoning can be done with eight beef or chicken bouillon cubes or the equivalent in granules. You can also season with one or two tablespoons dry onion soup mix instead of the bouillon. Vary the seasoning for effect. Take a VERY large soup kettle. Cut and chop all vegetables into small chunks. Boil in water with seasoning, plus salt and pepper to taste for about ten minutes. You may use a quart of water or more to start with. Lower heat after ten minutes and simmer until desired consistency of vegetables is reached. Increase or decrease water while cooking to get desired thickness or thinness of soup. This soup may be eaten at any time of the day.

If only three or four bowls are consumed daily, do not bother to count this into your daily ration of vegetables. Broccoli and/or mushrooms may be substituted in the recipe for cabbage, celery, or peppers if any of these are bothersome to you and your digestion.

For over four bowls (eight to twelve ounces of liquid) of soup per day, give up one fully cooked vegetable per bowl.

It is permitted to take about a quart of the Super Soup mixture after you have cooked it and place it in a crock pot with from two to four ounces of your daily allotment of beef, chicken, fish, seafood, turkey, lean pork, or lamb. Put the mixture of soup and protein and allow it to cook all day long, or all night long if you plan to carry it to work with you. Be creative in the use of spices and seasonings to enhance the flavor. The delicious stew, gumbo, or chowder produced will help suppress hunger during the day, or at night when you return home from work. Count the protein portion (beef, etc.) as part of your daily allowance and treat the soup as free food.

Dr. Cooper's Vidalia Onion Soup

Take 5 cups of thinly-sliced Vidalia onions. Other, inferior onions could be used, but the results will be less tasty. Do not use red onions at all! Also use 6 ounces of Butter Buds liquid, 1/2 teaspoon dry mustard, 1 quart of water or chicken stock, a dash of thyme, 1 tablespoon of Tamari soy sauce, 3 tablespoons dry white wine. Options to add also include 2 small crushed cloves of garlic, one envelope of Sweet'n Low, and salt to taste.

Cook the onions and optional garlic, if desired. Lightly sauté them, along with the 6 ounces of Butter Buds in a Teflon or Pam-coated skillet. Cook over medium heat until the onions begin to brown. Stir frequently with wooden spoon or spatula. Add mustard and thyme and mix in thoroughly. Empty the browned onion and spice mixture into a large saucepan. Add remaining ingredients. Cook slowly with pan covered for at least 30 minutes. Pour into oven-safe soup bowls. Sprinkle a light coating of grated cheese over each bowl after filling. Prior to serving you may want to place in an oven just long enough to melt the cheese. Best served with toasted Malsovit bread or the Malsovit Meal Wafers. Only one serving daily is allowed during the diet phase. Equal to 1/2 starch-bread portion.

These recipes are just possible ones you could use. They were developed by me or contributed by my patients. There are a lot of others out there that may be just as delicious and low in calories. Once you have attained your slimmer figure, you can experiment yourself and read the food magazines for low-Calorie food tips and recipes.

There are other recipes for low-calorie cooking in the Appendix section at the end of this book.

CHAPTER FIVE

BEHAVIOR MODIFICATION TECHNIQUES THAT WORK

In this chapter are over a hundred hints for you to look over. Not all will apply to your particular situation, but it is hoped that a substantial number of them will. We all live in a literal jungle of food cues and inducements to stray from a diet. We are bombarded from morning to night with food commercials, signs advertising food, food and beverages being consumed around us, and the temptations offered by feeders and other saboteurs, as you will read about in this book.

Read through this chapter a page or so at a time. Don't try to memorize or absorb all of it at once. See where the advice fits you, and try it. You will be pleased to see how often these little tricks work for you. They are not neatly organized into home, office, church, and social situations. I deliberately have fragmented them to induce you to look at only a few at a time.

The techniques that you read about for controlling your problem eating have been developed by psychologists and physicians over a period of three decades. Some ingenious research has gone into proving that some of them work. Most of those you see here were used by me when I was slimming down from 240 to 180 pounds back in 1967. The hints are numbered so that you can keep up with them, but number one hundred is just as important as number one. I hope you enjoy them as much as I have enjoyed using them and making them work for me.

ONE HUNDRED (MORE OR LESS) HINTS FOR StAYING OUT OF TROUBLE WHILE DIETING

1) Buy fresh or frozen vegetables if possible. Canned vegetables are loaded with sodium in most cases. It will help you avoid unwanted swelling, bloating, or edema. Learn to read and interpret the nutritional labels on food cans, bottles, cartons, and packages. Remember that most reputable food and beverage companies will list the nutritional composition.

The nutritional information per serving should include serving size, servings per package, percentage of U.S. Recommended Daily Allowances, and amounts of calories, protein, carbohydrate, fat, and sodium per serving.

2) When you have done well, and are losing fat steadily, reward yourself with a non-food treat. Buy a book you have wanted, get a new and smaller piece of clothing, go to a movie (no popcorn, please!), or have some other treat that doesn't involve eating or drinking.

3) Do not eat or drink while you are driving or riding in a car or other vehicle, unless it is an apple.

4) Do not eat or drink while watching television, listening to the radio, reading, or listening to tape or disc music. You should have no distractions when eating.

5) Avoid napping or dozing after a meal. Try and move around, either inside or outside your home. Take a short walk, but don't sit down in that recliner or stretch out on your bed until bedtime. Keep a record of your exercise for each day, even if it is just a short walk. This makes you think about exercise more and prevents the "Couch Potato Syndrome" in most cases. If you do not exercise, you must put down "NONE" in your daily diary.

6) Keep all sweets that you like out of your house. Tell your family that they are to get their sweets elsewhere, unless it is a sweet that you can't stand. I am absolutely turned off by licorice and chocolate mints, so I ask my family to keep those around but nothing else. Those two types of sweet are what I keep for Halloween Trick or Treaters. There's no temptation to eat them after the holiday is over.

Also, don't buy Girl Scout Cookies. It is better to give a contribution to this organization and tell them to keep their sweets to themselves. That way you aren't trapped in your home with cookies staring you in the face or calling to you from the kitchen at 3:00 A.M.

7) If you want something cold and sweet, get some Tupperware popsicle molds and make popsicles with sugar-free Kool-Aid or Crystal Light. Don't keep ice cream, ice milk, or frozen desserts in your home.

8) A bowl or cup of partially frozen orange or grapefruit juice with a tiny amount of gelatin added is sometimes enough to satisfy my sweet tooth. Pour the juice into a cup or bowl. Place in the freezer until it just begins to crystallize. Take it out and stir well. Enjoy!

9) Never go to the grocery store hungry. There are studies that tend to show that this prevents you from buying too much problem food. There are also studies that tend to show the opposite. I still feel it is better to have eaten prior to buying foods. I always bring a list and unless there is a special sale on something legal, I will not buy anything not on that paper. I only take enough money to buy what I NEED and not what I CRAVE!

10) Freeze leftovers or discard them. Problem foods that enter your house should never be saved. Use the leftover useful foods later when needed, but don't eat them now.

11) Use a distinctive placemat whenever you eat. Use a knife, spoon, and fork to eat whatever you are consuming, even if it is, heaven forbid, a candy bar. Set the table, put the candy bar on a plate and slowly eat it using your knife, spoon, and fork. Even at three in the morning, set your table if you want that Oreo cookie. Now, after all that, do you still want the cookie, or are you feeling a little bit ridiculous?

Some researchers feel that the externality theory of behavior modification is not valid, at least to the degree we once thought. It was once felt that the obese obey very little of the internal signals from their bodies but are mostly controlled by external cues and signals to eat (externality), based on their prior conditioning and experience. I frankly disagree, since I am often controlled by my environment and am tempted to indulge in problem eating.

12) Avoid "finger food" that is picked up in the hand, nibbled on, dipped into something, or simply is one bite per morsel. This type of food is deadly to a diet. You can consume an enormous amount of this type of food at a party or reception.

13) Stay away from most alcohol during the initial stages of your diet program. Alcohol may slow down your ability to burn fat while speeding up your ability to produce fatty tissue and decreasing your inhibitions and sense of control over your eating. It is no accident that the words, "Bon Appetit" are spoken as a pre-dinner alcoholic beverage is drunk.

14) Observe overweight people in restaurants and cafeterias. Be critical, as if you were a dietician or physician monitoring them. Do they shovel and pour the food in? Is this how you might look? Think about that the next time YOU are out and eating.

15) In your home set up a mirror in front of you at the table and see how you appear as you eat. Is it pleasant for you to see yourself eating, or does something disturb you about your eating habits?

16) Use a tiny cocktail fork to eat with. Cut your meat and other foods into tinier bites. Eat slowly and see if you aren't eating less. Chopsticks are also another way to slow down your eating.

17) Eat soup or salad before every lunch and dinner meal. Eat slowly, using a teaspoon for the soup and a cocktail fork for the salad. Try and make both last twice as long as your previous time. There DOES seem to be a delay factor of about 20 minutes from the time eating starts until the brain "knows" it is satisfied. This is for patients of normal weight. If the obese are not sensitive to internal signals, does the tactic have validity? It seems to, at least in my practice, so perhaps there is a certain amount of dual signal sensitivity in an overweight person.

18) Use a small salad plate instead of a regular-sized dinner plate and see if the same size portion doesn't look larger. Better still, put even smaller portions on the smaller salad plate. Visual signals are powerful ones for the obese, both to turn on and turn off eating at certain times.

19) If you are invited to a party, call your hostess up and explain that you are having problems with certain foods. They don't agree with you (they break you out in fat!), and you would like very much to come, but you didn't want to hurt her feelings by appearing to not like the food if it is one of your problem items. See if she can suggest something else for you to eat, or maybe you will be lucky and there will be nothing but "diet food" there at the function. Most hosts and hostesses are cooperative and helpful if they are given an opportunity. This is also a good exercise in the use of assertiveness for the patient. Using Cognitive Restructuring (CR) techniques, as covered later in this book, the person can practice "being good" in his or her mind for a few times before actually making the call.

20) At a party, arrive late and leave early if possible. Have something to eat, even if it is just an apple, before you get there. Sit down somewhere far away from the dips, peanuts, chips, and other high-calorie snacks and finger foods. Get yourself a non-caloric drink and sit down and enjoy the other guests. If it is a buffet, get at the end of the line and get TWO items. Eat them and then go back and get ONE with each subsequent trip until the party is over. If you do it correctly, everyone will wonder why you are losing when you are "eating so much." You have only given the appearance of eating a lot, but it satisfies your hostess.

21) Avoid food-related functions at the church or synagogue. Find out, if you must attend, whether the food is being served before or after the function. If before, come in late. If after, get out of there as soon as it is polite to do so. Politely turn down food offered to you, usually by some sweet old grandmotherly feeder, and say that it doesn't agree with you. See the reference to Feeders and Saboteurs later on in this book.

22) If you are going to be in an unavoidable situation where it appears you will have to eat a lot, save up some of your food portions over the three days prior to the wedding, anniversary, birthday party, or whatever. You may save ahead and build up a food portion balance, but may not "owe" yourself after the fact and promise to cut down the next few days. Those promises are meant at the time but are hard to keep.

23) When the craving for sweets is at its worse, use a portion of fruit. Cut the fruit up with a knife and eat one tiny morsel of it at a time. Feel the texture and taste of the fruit in your mouth. Chew each bite slowly and carefully, letting the taste buds get the full effect of each bite. Let each bite be a sensuous experience. Drink liberal amounts of fluids after each bite is swallowed.

24) When you are just about to raid the refrigerator or pantry for something to eat, get out of the house, or at least the kitchen. Take a walk or do some yard work. Find some task to do and tell yourself that you MIGHT have some of whatever it is, but first you are going to wait 30 minutes before you have it. If you last 30 minutes, go for a full hour. Keep occupying yourself until the impulse goes away or until an actual mealtime or bedtime comes.

25) Any time between meals that you want a forbidden snack, brush your teeth or use mouthwash. This technique works for either eating or smoking problems. It is better if the mouthwash is one that is slightly tart or astringent, such as Lavoris.

26) Keep your scale in the kitchen, not in the bathroom. Weigh yourself as often as you need to: when you need reinforcement. or when you know that stepping on the scale will stop you from a binge. Remember that all your weight is NOT fat. If the scales show a loss, believe them. If there is no WEIGHT loss, but you are staying on your program, look for changes in the way clothing fits. If your clothes fit looser, it probably means that you are losing FAT. This is one of the hardest things to explain to a patient. The body fat content is decreasing, the protein content is increasing from exercise, the content of water is fluctuating, and the weight may vary greatly from one day to the next. It is important for you to be aware of what is going on in your body, or there will be a certain amount of disgust and discouragement at the "weight gain" on the scales.

27) Buy a kitchen timer. Set it for 10 minutes whenever you want to eat and it's not mealtime. Take that 10-minute pause to think through whether or not you really want, or need, to eat. It could be that another form of recreation or amusement would be just as satisfying. Delay tactics are powerful in preventing impulse eating. With enough delays there may be a diminution or extinguishing of the impulse to snack or nibble.

28) At mealtime, set the timer for 20 minutes. Always try to stretch out mealtimes for at least that long. Studies show that it takes about 20 minutes for your brain to become aware that the stomach is full and you are "satisfied." Setting a timer will let you cue into your body's sense of true hunger. This is another reference to the 20 minutes theory. I find that even if it is not totally accurate to say the above, it works in practice for me and my patients.

29) Jot down into a notebook, or use a diary sheet, everything you eat, how you feel when you eat, and the person(s) you're with, and review it at day's end. That way, you can readily associate the triggering incidents, feelings, and people that might be leading you to eat too much. Being forewarned is being prepared and less vulnerable.

30) Eat in one established place at home to eliminate all other environmental clues. This sort of routine can eliminate the absent-minded eating in front of the TV, in the den while reading, or in the kitchen while talking on the phone. Automatic eating is a real entity and flourishes best where the awareness level of the patient is low.

31) Make eating a pleasure. Take your time and enjoy each bite. Put out your distinctive place setting. Use cut flowers or candles if you like. Making eating enjoyable is a sure way to help get rid of negative feelings about your diet. The more you enjoy eating, the more in control of your diet you can be, and the more successful you can become at losing unwanted pounds forever.

32) Wrap your tiny eating utensils in a cloth napkin so that the start of a meal is a deliberate moment. What you are introducing to the eating process is the making of a conscious decision, which will help you take responsibility for what you eat. Doing that will also slow you down so that you begin eating after everyone else does, another good habit to follow.

33) Eat with your right hand if you are left-handed and vice versa. The awkwardness will slow your eating pace as well as help you appreciate the tastes and textures of food. This is almost as good as using chopsticks.

34) Eat your favorite foods first at meals, so that when you begin to feel full, you won't be as reluctant to stop eating as you would if that food were still on your plate.

35) When you are served a much larger than desired portion of food at a restaurant, push away half the food and pepper or salt it heavily. By doing so, you are heading off the temptation to continue eating, even when you feel full, just because someone else decided on the portion size for you and without your approval. A lot of people are either "depression babies," or their parents are. To waste food is a cardinal sin for them. It may be impossible for them to "ruin" food like this, but they can still take the leftovers home and freeze or refrigerate them for later use.

36) Another trick is to oversalt the remaining food on your plate when you begin to feel full. This is almost the same thing as the previous hint, but is somewhat different if you think about it.

37) Put your eating utensils down after every third bite. Pause and enjoy what you are chewing.

38) Suck on, but do NOT chew, ice chips when you are cooking, so that you don't taste or nibble. You can take in an incredible amount of calories if you taste while cooking a meal. You can also drink extra amounts of cold water while cooking.

39) If you are an incurable "taster" during cooking and the previous suggestions didn't work, try wearing a surgical mask over your mouth, or a bandanna that may make you look like a stagecoach robber in a western movie. Either one will make you aware of how many times that stirring spoon or fork comes up to your mouth with food on it. The spoon or fork will bump against the mask and make you aware of this unconscious tasting and nibbling. Most hardware and building supply stores have these types of masks for use when a workman is sanding or working around dust.

40) Use small half-cup measuring cups to serve food from pots and pans directly to the plate. Never put food on the table family-style. It is too easy to get another helping.

41) Carry little packets of low-calorie salad dressing with you to use in restaurants or at dinner parties, or only have lemon juice or vinegar on salads. Both Walden Farms and Estee/DiaMel have a line of the individual servings of salad dressing, but there may be some more companies who also market these convenient packets. Use oil-free dressings when you can.

42) You can also ask your druggist for a two-ounce bottle with a screw cap. Fill it from a large bottle of diet dressing and carry it in your purse, pocket, or briefcase. Take it along with you when you eat out.

43) Read package labels and know the difference between similar foods. For example, unflavored yogurt has no added sugar. Patients see the "low-fat" part of the label, but don't take the time to fully read the label and notice the extra sugar on flavored yogurt containers. If you want flavored yogurt, use the ones that have added Nutrasweet instead of sugar. Most have 90 to 110 calories per serving, with Yoplait, Kroger, and Light N' Lively having these as I write this chapter.

44) Be aware of serving sizes. For example, the smallest container (8 ounces) of cottage cheese, which many women eat for lunch, is two servings, not one. Cottage cheese also varies in content of fat and calorie count. One low-fat cottage cheese contains 90 calories and 1 gram of fat per serving. Another cottage cheese made with milk with greater fat content has 120 calories and 5 grams of fat per serving.

45) Some of the preceding hints came from *Nutritioning Parents,* a government publication. There are a lot of good sources of nutritional information available from the federal, state, and county governmental agencies, not to mention the Heart Association, the Cancer Society, and other groups. Take advantage of the tremendous amount of circulating knowledge that is largely free for the asking or can be had with a small donation.

46) Don't set yourself up for failure in dieting. If you don't buy it, don't accept it from someone else, or don't allow it to enter your home, you won't eat it. It has to be there first, or you can't eat or drink it. Ask your family to help you by getting them to read the open letter in another chapter of this book.

47) When eating out, be sure and tell the server what you want. Don't let yourself be intimidated by the waiter. If you want an entree without sauce, or with sauce on the side, tell him. If you want something left off the plate, let the waiter know ahead of time to omit that item. If it is brought anyhow, ask the waiter to take the plate back and remove the offending item. If you let it sit on your plate, you may nibble on it or eat all of it.

48) Get out of your office when your co-workers start bringing out the snacks or the birthday cake and ice cream. Go and wish the other person a happy birthday, happy retirement, etc., but don't let anyone hand you a plate of goodies. Put your hands behind your back and smile, but do not offer to accept it. Use the parrot technique that is discussed elsewhere in this book. Continue to smile and agreeably refuse with the same phrase: "No thank you, I just don't care for it." I always warn my patients to never admit they are dieting. They just simply don't care for whatever is being offered.

49) Instead of staying in your office during lunch and eating (and sharing the wrong foods with others), go outside if the weather permits. Take a walk and get away from your work environment for a while.

50) Get a set routine for meals and permitted snacks. Try and set up a natural body rhythm that will take hunger, exercise, sleep, and other activities into consideration. Let your routine be your support and protection against problem eating.

51) Avoid bars and pubs for a while until you are a lot stronger than you might be now. Try not to drink, but if you do, drink moderately and concentrate on using diluted drinks ($\frac{1}{2}$ jigger of spirits in 12 to 16 ounces of mixer, one ounce of dry wine in 12 ounces of soda) or drink lite beer from a jigger glass instead of a mug or can or bottle.

52) If you go into a bar, remember to avoid the salty chips, peanuts, and popcorn. They are there to make you thirsty for several more drinks. Always drink alcohol AFTER a meal, never on an empty stomach. Alcoholic drinks before dinner tend to make you eat and drink more. This advice is obviously for after you are on maintenance. Avoid alcohol in all forms while trying to lose weight.

53) You may be out with a group that has ordered a wine to share among you. Have a half-glass and let it sit there after the first small sip. If you empty your glass, it gets filled again. If you do not empty it, you will not have to refuse refills. Be sure there is some other type of beverage on the table, with water as the preferred drink.

You can also turn your glass upside down before the wine is opened.

54) Tonic water, club soda, diet drinks, plain water, mineral water, orange juice, grapefruit juice, and tomato juice are usually in a bar or restaurant. Get one of these drinks in these places, or at a party. It looks like you are drinking and if it makes you uncomfortable to be seen without something in your hand, these make good alternative choices instead of alcoholic drinks.

55) Try to make breakfast the biggest meal of your day. If you are not used to eating breakfast, start off slowly and add food gradually over a period of a week. You can also go to bed without supper one night. The next morning you WILL eat. Eat like a king at breakfast, like a squire at lunch, and like a peasant at night. Make your first two meals of the day contain over half of your calories for the day, perhaps even as much as two-thirds.

56) Make yourself do work to get your food. Don't have someone else get it for you. Get up and get it yourself. If you do get something, only get a little bit of it and leave the kitchen. Researchers have shown that the lack of immediate contact with food, even if it is only in the next room, is enough to slow or stop extra food intake in many cases.

57) The usual bout of "hunger" will last for less than 30 minutes. If you delay your eating, the chances are that time and a few antacid tablets will abort the desire to eat. This IS one cue that is internal and could be mistaken for hunger. The rebound of hydrochloric acid secretion about two hours after a meal can sometimes make a person "hungry" because of the sensation of emptiness, gnawing, or actual pain in the pit of the stomach. Food relieves the problem, but with a price of added caloric intake. Antacids in liquid or tablet form may do the same job of relieving discomfort, without a penalty of extra calories.

58) Don't skip meals. There is nothing more futile than getting unrealistic and skipping meals to "lose faster." In fact, cutting your daily food intake down may actually slow you down in fat loss. You might stop burning as much fat and start cannibalizing your own body protein, and that is not such a good idea. Eat everything that is prescribed for you on your diet. If there is a problem with that instruction, see your therapist and ask for help in working it out.

59) The other side of the coin on skipping meals is that the person will omit certain necessary foods and replace them with problem foods. This is another sure way to fail. Don't swap "apples" for "oranges" on your diet program.

60) Try and make sure that, with the exception of foods prepared for the present meal, there are no easily cooked, or ready-to-eat foods in the house. If there is a delay in getting the food because of the necessity to prepare or cook it, the chances are that you might lose the urge long before the snack is ready for you. This is more of the Externality Theory in action, and it seems to work. Food or beverages that can't be picked up, put in the mouth, and swallowed will not be consumed. Be careful not to offer every excuse possible, including the need to keep the children and spouse supplied with snacks. You must counter this tendency with logic and reason with yourself that most of the problem foods taken home will be consumed by you, and not the family, if it stays there.

61) Never eat standing up or lying down.

62) Avoid secret or closet eating. Have someone who is sympathetic and helpful around if you have decided to eat a problem food.

63) Leave the table immediately after you have finished. Do not remain to watch others eat. There is nothing sacred about someone sitting at the table because of another person's slow eating.

64) Have your family clear their own plates directly into the garbage or disposal. Don't let food sit around. You might go back to the table and nibble.

65) Keep your food in containers that are opaque and impossible to see into. Visual cues sometimes trigger eating, too.

66) Never buy goodies for your family because you will wind up eating a good percentage of what you bring home. Let your family go off without you for treats. Never take your children to a problem food location, such as a pizza parlor, hamburger stand, frozen yogurt store, Mexican restaurant, or candy store.

67) Never take your child to the grocery store. It is cheaper to hire someone, or swap services with another mother, so that the child is cared for while you shop. Children are bombarded with TV ads for junk food and will tirelessly pester you to buy these foods while you are trying to pick out the right things for your family.

68) Try and stay out of food ruts. Vary the types of the different foods and the ways they are cooked. Boredom is one of your worst enemies. Spices, such as those mentioned in another chapter, add almost no calories to a dish but make it interesting and tasty.

69) When eating out, do a little pre-planning before you go. Visualize yourself, using CR, at the restaurant. Imagine how you will order your food and how you will tell what your preferences are. Refuse desserts for now. You will have some later on your maintenance program, but it is better to stay away from these highly concentrated sweets until you are a lot stronger in your habit patterns.

70) Skip the bread, butter, chips, pre-dinner drinks and other traps. Ask for a glass of mineral water, or some other harmless beverage, and refuse to get any bread out of the basket. If your restaurant is really service-minded, the waiter may actually put bread on your bread plate for you. This can be some Malsovit bread that you have brought with you in a baggy. A hand held over the plate is an assertive way to say no without offending. The same for your wine glass. Turn it upside down or cover it with your hand when the wine steward comes around.

71) Be careful to trim off fats and brush off fatty and creamy sauces from your foods. Carefully trim off the skin and fat from poultry before eating the inner meats.

72) You can ask for "seconds" on vegetable items and salads, but make sure the Hollandaise sauce and the fatty salad dressings are served on the side. It will appear that you are eating a lot, but actually you are eating foods with low densities as far as calories are concerned.

73) Avoid chocolate milk and whole milk as beverages when possible. Use skim milk and products made from lower-fat milk.

74) A fruit cup for dessert is a good choice, but make sure it is fresh fruit. Fruit canned in heavy syrup, or in any syrup at all, is loaded with sugar. In fact, the word syrup refers to sugar dissolved in water.

75) The words "light" and "diet" are seen a lot on certain foodstuff packages. Also, low-calorie and low-fat are seen frequently. These words, in themselves, mean little. Something can be low-fat, as yogurt and frozen yogurt are, and still be loaded with empty sugar calories.

76) Keep some sort of daily diary that matches your routine. The feedback between you and yourself is a powerful influence on eating. If your therapist sees it too, the feedback loop is extended and strengthened. The paper you write the diary details on becomes magic paper. All you have to do is write down what you eat and you help yourself lose weight faster. The Cooper Charts are excellent ways to keep track of your food intake, both during the weight loss phase and in the maintenance period. Information about ordering the charts is at the very back of this book.

77) It is almost a rule in obesity treatment: if you don't walk, you don't lose. The body is capable of fighting you through the set point mechanism and can frustrate your efforts to lose fat. Walking seems to bypass this set point and the weight loss continues, in spite of the interference by the body. Make it a point to walk every day, no matter what. It is possible to do other exercises as an alternative if walking is difficult or impossible for a person. See the chapter on exercise for other information.

78) This hint is also to tell you to walk. The natural tendency of the overweight person is to be less active. Overweight persons will kill to avoid walking, in fact; there have been fatal fights in parking lots over a space that was 50 feet closer to a department store entrance than another equally good space (in GOOD weather).

79) Don't be a "Couch Potato" and sit all the time. Move around and keep your body healthy and your calorie consumption up. Wear athletic clothes and use them. Don't be like one of my patients that I observed one afternoon at a local shopping center. She is not handicapped, but she drove right up to the front of a store, parked in the handicapped space, and bounced into the store wearing her tennis outfit. The weather was good and there was a parking space only 100 feet away from where she parked.

80) If it is appropriate in your life style, stay sexually active. "Use it or lose it" is not an idle statement. This fact is a part of adult life for the majority of us. Unless there is a problem with

your spouse or partner, try to be as active as you were at your prime. We often replace sex with food, an unnatural and tragic situation. Even fairly heavy men and women can enjoy active and fulfilling sex lives. There are competent counselors to help with mechanical or psychological problems. Love is an important thing in everyone's life, and intimacy should not be ignored.

81) Be realistic about what you can expect to lose every month. Don't be upset about fluctuations in weight as a result of fluid retention or healthy muscle growth. If your activity pattern allows for two or three pounds of fat loss a week, consider yourself lucky. Only in science fiction stories, or certain diet books, do we find the ten-pounds-a-week stories and claims. It is physically impossible for most of us to lose more than eight to ten pounds a month. Our bodies just won't let go of much more than that.

82) There are advantages to letting some of your real friends know you are dieting. Let these good friends help you, but beware of feeders and saboteurs. Don't let them know you are trying to lose fat.

83) When you are at the end of your work day and are tired, hungry, angry, anxious, provoked, and perhaps a dozen other things too, stop for a minute before entering your home. Plan to have something, such as a tuna salad or fruit plate, waiting on you when you first step in the door. My Super Soup is another good idea for your homecoming snack. Stop for a minute before you enter your home and visualize yourself having a snack at your table with the placemat and the rest of your place setting in front of you. Avoid going by a fast food restaurant on the way home and getting something to go. While sitting in your office at the end of the day, visualize yourself going straight home. Use this technique to avoid impulse buys of problem foods.

84) Reward yourself with a soothing hot bath when you have had your snack. Luxuriate in the water and let the heat soak into your body, carrying away all the soreness and the muscle spasms in the neck and the upper back. Feel the tension leaving your body as every muscle in your body relaxes. Your body is now relaxed. It doesn't require problem foods to cover up your nervousness or tension. You can now eat what you NEED, rather than what you CRAVED. You can look forward to a good night's sleep and waking up the next morning refreshed and alert. These mental images can be real to you if you let them. Treat yourself to a hot bath as a reward for a hard day's work.

85) Put some other barrier between you and food. Try and polish your nails when you are hungry. Another tactic is to find something dirty and grubby to do that will make your hands so filthy that you would not eat at that time. I often dig in my flower garden whenever the urge to eat hits me. Perhaps the cellar, basement, or attic needs a good cleaning. Unless you have hidden the Oreo cookies there, you are probably safe.

86) Another hint about preventing tasting while cooking: use sugar-free chewing gum and chew it the whole time you are cooking a meal. You can also nibble on something benign such as celery. Cut the celery into small chunks. Chew the celery pieces, but chew them well. Make each chunk last at least three or four minutes.

87) For night eaters, keep some antacid by the bedside, along with a glass of skim milk and a piece of fruit. Account for the food with your Cooper Charts (one white and one orange portion) during the day and save these for bedtime. You might also think about buying one of the several refrigerator alarms that have been offered lately. It wakes up the rest of the family and may deter you from raiding the refrigerator.

88) Put encouraging messages around the house, particularly in the kitchen, on the pantry door, on the refrigerator, and at work. Let them say whatever you want them to. Some that I have used are listed below:

A minute in the mouth, an hour in the stomach,
and a lifetime on the hips.
A waist is a terrible thing to mind.
Do you really need that? Be honest now!

89) Find a kindred spirit who is also dieting and get support from each other. Speak to this person or persons every day if possible. Encourage each other. Try and walk daily with this person. It pays off for both of you in increased fat loss. This mutual support works in obesity, just as it works in alcoholism. When you diet, you diet ALONE! That is, you do unless you seek out the support you need from others with the same problem. Overeaters Anonymous is often a worthwhile source of help for dieters.

90) Avoid negative people. Divorce yourself from those who would hinder your progress through their own problems in dealing with life.

91) Think thin. Visualize yourself as a thin person with a healthy body and boundless energy. See yourself in thin clothes and outfits.

92) Learn to be assertive with others and yourself. Being assertive means letting your needs be known in a non-aggressive way. It doesn't mean that you have to be rude or obnoxious, just firm.

93) Leave something on your plate with every meal. Refuse to clean your plate. Your leaving something won't keep someone in Cambodia from starving. Get rid of your ideas about waste. What's the biggest waste — eating everything and compromising your diet, or leaving a little bit and not eating it? The answer is obvious.

94) Try and get your grocer or delicatessen worker to weigh out things for you in three-ounce or four-ounce packages and separately wrap them for you. Portion control starts in the store. Use smaller cans, rather than the larger and more wasteful sizes. Buy leaner cuts of meat. They are not Prime or Choice grades, but they are lower in fat and this makes it easier for you to practice calorie control by cutting back on the high-fat meats.

95) Practice delays during a meal. Deliberately place your utensils on the table and relax for a moment. Try and wait a minute or more before starting to eat again. Use these delays to build confidence in your ability to control your environment, rather than having it control you.

96) If you are in a restaurant and have ordered a standard entree that is too much for you to eat, don't hesitate to take the remainder home rather than just eating another four ounces of filet or other dish. Don't be embarrassed to ask for help from the waiter.

97) Avoid the temptation to "lose weight" by taking excessively strong laxatives and probably unneeded diuretics (water pills). These have their price in side-effects and are not benign in their actions. Watch and make sure that your fiber and fluid intake is high enough to help with regularity without the need for laxatives. The other thing required for regularity is walking. It is extremely rare to see an active walker who has bowel problems. They just don't have them much. The need for diuretics can also be bypassed by making sure the sodium intake is low enough and that the water intake is sufficient.

98) Don't expect miracles. It takes hard work to get down to a slim weight and figure. There is no shortcut in the process. Your habits, your thinking, your eating, and your activity pattern must all change, or the entire process is futile. The good news is that it really isn't that hard to do. The whole thing boils down to making a lot of small changes in your life.

99) Look upon this entire program of weight loss as a learning situation. You are learning a skill and you may make mistakes along the way. Don't be punitive with yourself. Be tolerant and forgiving of yourself and others. Expect to have difficulties and be ready for them. When mistakes or problems arise, look upon them as golden opportunities to show what you can do to excel at the task of slimming yourself.

100) Never go shopping or run errands with another woman, unless she is a saint. Most shopping and errand trips wind up in some caloric den of iniquity and you can be trapped by even a well-meaning person who ISN'T on a diet.

101) The last suggestion I have for you is to be just a little bit cautious and slightly paranoid in your daily dealings with all those who might offer you food or trigger problem eating in you. Don't trust anyone. Dieters are natural targets of feeders and saboteurs. Remember again that just because you are paranoid doesn't mean that everyone isn't against you!

Read these items over, along with your other literature and work toward controlling your life, instead of the reverse situation. Good luck in your quest for a slimmer body.

CHAPTER SIX

VITAMINS AND MINERALS

Vitamins and minerals are a much misunderstood group of nutritional substances. They have been damned for being worthless or dangerous, and praised for being the means for curing all ills, psychic, physical, and metaphysical. Few nutritionists on either side of the Atlantic will disagree that if the proper kinds of foods are consumed every day in the correct quantities, there is no real need for vitamins and minerals to be taken as supplements.

It is also almost universally agreed that when the diet contains less than 1,200 to 1,400 Calories a day, the need for supplementation with an intelligent quantity of vitamins and minerals becomes more critical. In the interest of practicality, and because of the increased metabolic and chemical workload placed on the body during the weight loss, it becomes a practical and reasonable measure to get *at least* what is calculated to be the minimum daily requirement for each of these substances to avoid any short-term or long-term problems with deficiency states.

You and your physician will decide whether or not you require these supplements. Each case is different and must be decided on an individual basis. Vitamins and minerals act as catalysts or co-factors in the hundreds of different chemical reactions that are essential to life. They are a group of so-called "chemical helpers" that speed up and intensify the biochemical machinery in each of our bodies.

When you, as a slimmer or dieter, take one or more supplements on your doctor's orders, you are insuring that nothing goes wrong with your body chemistry as a result of a deficiency. It is a prudent thing to do in most cases. I usually recommend a therapeutic multiple vitamin, without iron and other minerals, since these must be dispensed in a child-proof bottle to avoid ingestion of iron and other potentially toxic items in the formula. You may wish to review what I consider an ideal slimmer's vitamin formula at the end of this chapter.

You may know a lot about nutritional supplements, or you may know virtually nothing. In order to place each one in perspective, I have listed each one, along with some information about it. I am ignoring some of the more bizarre claims made by some "experts," both in and out of the medical field. The only ones I am very cautious about are vitamins A and D, along with iron. These three substances have been the cause of a lot of grief over the years from unintentional or deliberate overdosing. The medical literature is full of cases of toxicity and poisoning from poor judgement or accidents. The others have been attacked occasionally but are safe in normal doses.

VITAMIN A

This vitamin is intimately connected with the many processes involving the lining cells of the body, including the skin, the eyes, the lining of the bronchial tree, and other similar lining or epithelial structures. It is also involved in the metabolism of fat and in the processes of vision, particularly night vision. A generous amount of vitamin A is obtained from liver, milk, eggs, butter, and vegetables (both dark green leafy vegetables and yellow vegetables), and fruit. Those fruits and vegetables high in vitamins A and C are listed in a previous chapter.

Vitamins A and C, plus zinc, have also been noted to assist in the building of collagen (connective tissue) and other proteins in nutritionally depleted states. Vitamin A can also cause toxicity if taken in excess amounts.

VITAMIN B-1

Thiamine, or vitamin B-1, is one of the most important vitamins in fat and sugar metabolism. In one step in the metabolism of sugar (glucose) a substance called pyruvate has to be changed to acetate, or the reaction for getting energy from simple carbohydrates cannot continue. Fortunately for us, thiamine helps speed up this reaction, along with a few similar ones, and the process of aerobic energy production in the cells is continued at an optimal rate.

Doctors used to see a lot of a B-1 deficiency state known as beriberi, but this is virtually unknown now. Thiamine is found in wheat germ, whole grain bread, nuts, legumes, brown rice and rice bran, asparagus, okra, leafy green vegetables, and prunes.

VITAMIN B-2

Riboflavin, or vitamin B-2, plays a pivotal role in the metabolism and energy balance of the body in the handling of fats, proteins, and carbohydrates. It is a major vitamin. In order to oxidize the foodstuffs we consume for energy, there must be a certain chain of chemical events or reactions occurring. Both riboflavin and niacin (B-3) must be present and utilized in the cell for the body to oxidize the food materials. To illustrate just how important this energy (hydrogen transport) chain is, if a substance like cyanide is introduced into the body and this energy chain is blocked, the person dies quickly.

By taking adequate amounts of B-2 we can insure that the oxidation processes in the body continue at the needed rapid rate and there is no slowdown caused by these relative deficiencies. Some of the same sources for B-1 are also good ones for B-2. These include milk, liver, whole grain bread, leafy green vegetables, legumes, okra, avocado, Brussels sprouts, and dried prunes and apricots.

VITAMIN B-3

Niacin (nicotinic acid) and niacinamide (nicotinamide) are both active as B-3 and the body can use either for its purposes. The oxidative chemical chain involved in energy metabolism is also assisted by this vitamin. These energy-producing reactions are vitally important when large amounts of body fat are burned for energy. A relative lack of B-3 might be the cause of a slowdown in energy metabolism and, therefore, in the rate of fat loss. Yeast, lean meats, liver, wheat and rice bran, kelp, whole grain bread, mushrooms, apricots, and prunes are several good sources, as are some leafy green vegetables.

Niacin, but not niacinamide, can cause an intense flushing over the skin of the upper body after it is taken in certain dosage strengths. This is caused by a release of histamine from some of the body's cells and is harmless. Niacin is used to help control cholesterol levels and has some moderate effect in that role.

If you have a history of peptic ulcer, liver disease, jaundice, or gallbladder disease, use niacin only with your therapist's knowledge and consent. If you are on certain blood pressure drugs that are called "Beta blockers," be careful of episodes of low blood pressure that might result from taking additional niacin along with these medications.

VITAMIN B-6

Pyridoxine, or vitamin B-6, is primarily a vitamin of protein and amino acid metabolism but enters into other reactions as well. It is a vitamin intimately involved in certain important reactions that help change certain building blocks of protein, the amino acids, into other forms through a process called transamination.

Sources for this vitamin are similar to other B-Complex factors and there is rarely an absolute deficiency of pyridoxine as such. It has been found to be involved in some way with the metabolism of certain circulating hormones of the body and, according to *anecdotal* accounts, with the relief of the effects of the so-called "premenstrual syndrome." Some women who have a cyclic buildup of excessive hormone levels, along with all the problems connected with this syndrome, have reported that B-6 has helped them.

No one is quite sure how or why this comes about, or if there is only a placebo effect, but we do know that women who take as much as 50 to 100 mg. four times a day report beneficial effects. The diuresis, or release of excess and unwanted fluid retained by the body, is found in the absence of prescription diuretics and only seems to require the intake of an excess amount of water and the B-6 for the relief to be obtained.

Recent medical reports mention neurological disorders associated with massive amounts of B-6, usually at doses of over 600 mg. daily, but there have been no reports of similar problems in the doses mentioned above of 400 mg. a day or less.

VITAMIN C

Ascorbic acid, or vitamin C, has many known benefits and effects. While many are disputed, there are some that are definitely agreed on by all authorities. The benefits to the connective tissue and related structures through the actions of vitamin C have been documented for centuries, beginning with the prevention of scurvy by supplementing the diet with citrus fruits (limes, etc.).

There are certain chemical processes involving oxidation and reduction of foodstuffs that must have vitamin C to proceed properly. When connective tissue and the small capillaries supplying the cells of the body do not get Vitamin C, there is a tendency for the structure and function of these cells to become deranged. If this goes on long enough and there is either a relative or absolute lack of C, then scurvy results.

Sources for ascorbic acid include acerola, guava, peppers, citrus fruits, leafy green vegetables, and berries. Acerola is probably the richest source, with over 1,300 mg. of C per 100 gm. of juice or whole fruit.

VITAMIN D

The group of compounds that make up the different forms of vitamin D are chiefly responsible for the regulation of calcium and phosphorus metabolism in the body. There is very little deficiency of this vitamin in adults and children who drink milk and who get a reasonable amount of sunlight. Those with milk sensitivity and those who live in less temperate climates should probably supplement their food intake with extra D.

VITAMIN E

Vitamin E comes in several different forms, but particularly the d-alpha tocopherol seems to benefit our body the most. It is a controversial vitamin with many claims made for it, but it appears to have some action as an anti-oxidant and "cell healer" if anecdotal data is to be believed. Its actions on "restless leg syndrome" and on cystic mastitis of the breast seem real and reproducible enough. It may help prevent recurrences of thrombophlebitis and there may be some action in the healing of burns, but this is still unproven.

Whether or not E could be a help for you is uncertain. Ask your physician for his or her opinion. It doesn't seem to have toxicity in doses of 800 units daily in divided doses.

CALCIUM

It has been known for many years that calcium is necessary for the daily repair of our bones and joints. Bone tissue is being continually torn down by the body and replaced with new bone tissue. This process of breakdown and buildup is usually balanced, but in older women and men there is a gradual slowdown in the repair process and the bones become less dense, producing osteoporosis. The name refers to the decreased density and increased porosity of the bone structure.

Patients with osteoporosis are more likely to have painful joints and fractures of what become fragile bony tissue surfaces. There is also a tendency for the spine to become bent and distorted as the spinal column becomes less strong, giving in to gravity and muscle spasms. The result is the "little old lady or man" with a bent back and creaking joints.

The results described above are caused by neglect of good nutrition and a relative lack of dietary calcium. Where there is a milk product intolerance, consumption of calcium-rich vegetables and/or a proprietary calcium and vitamin D tablet is a prudent thing.

Dr. Martin Lipkin, of the Memorial Sloan-Kettering Cancer Center in New York, has published a research study indicating that supplemental dietary calcium has the effect of restoring normality to lining cells of the large intestine (colon). This restoration from an often pre-cancerous condition of the colon cells apparently reduces the risk of cancer of the colon. The risk reduction is apparently related to the protection that calcium gives from the irritant effect of bile and fatty acids on the lining cells.

COPPER

Copper is involved in many important enzyme systems in the body, including those that form several types of connective tissue and those that assist the body in processing iron into hemoglobin. It is needed only in very small amounts and can be toxic. There are, in fact, several serious disease states caused by excess copper deposition in body tissues. Copper also participates in a chemical pathway for the formation of certain pigments in the skin.

IRON

Iron is necessary as a component in the synthesis of hemoglobin and is active in certain other enzyme systems of the body. It is one of the most commonly deficient in the United States and the United Kingdom. This is particularly true in patients with poor diets or those with medical illnesses or physiological derangements that result in excessive blood loss (gastrointestinal bleeding, excess menstruation, etc.).

Iron is a common source of poisoning, with a relatively high mortality rate from overdoses. It should be used only if there is an indication to do so (low hemoglobin and iron levels), not just to "increase energy" in the body. The lack of energy could be coming from some other medical or psychological problem.

MAGNESIUM

Of all the elements in the body, magnesium has the most to do with the enzyme reactions necessary for life and health. Magnesium is the second most prevalent metallic ion in the cells of the body, with only potassium having a greater concentration. It is often lost, along with potassium, when patients take prescription diuretics. It is necessary for the proper functioning of the chemical systems involved in the synthesis and handling of proteins, fats, and carbohydrates in the body.

Magnesium, zinc, and manganese can be obtained from adequate amounts of eggs, green vegetables, mushrooms, lean meats and other protein-rich foods, dairy products, liver, other organ meats (high in fat, however), raisins, prunes, nuts, and whole grain breads.

MANGANESE

Many of the enzyme reactions that are related to glucose metabolism, energy production, and the synthesis or cartilage connective tissue are dependent on the presence of manganese to make them work properly. Deficiencies are rare. See magnesium, above, for good sources of manganese.

ZINC

Zinc is one of the most valuable metals classified as a trace element. It is involved in the formation of collagen, an important connective tissue component of the body, and in its use in the healing process after surgery or injury. It is also important in the formation of insulin and in the enzyme systems that control the acid-base balance of the body.

Zinc is often used preoperatively and after surgery to help healing occur faster. Zinc can be toxic, but the most common problems seen with zinc use are diarrhea and cramping following excessive intake.

Vitamins and minerals may be useful in your individual case. Be conservative for the best results. It is rare that you will require much more than the officially recommended daily amounts of any of them. I have found that the formula listed below has all the vitamins needed for daily use while on the Dutch Diet. It seems to give optimal support for this type of diet.

MULTIPLE VITAMIN FORMULA

Each tablet or capsule should contain:

Vitamin A - 5,000 units
Vitamin B-1 - 5 mg.
Vitamin B-2 - 5 mg.
Vitamin B-6 - 2 mg.
Vitamin B-12 - 4 mcg.
Vitamin C - 100 mg.
Vitamin D - 400 units
Calcium Pantothenate - 10 mg.
Niacinamide - 30 mg.

Where the minimum requirement has been established, the above formula exceeds this amount. Where there is no set requirement, the amount listed above is adequate by estimates of nutritionists and biochemists. The needs for daily mineral intake, particularly zinc and iron, are so different that no minerals were included, and it is hoped that the foodstuffs listed in the diet and maintenance chapters will be consumed as part of the respective diets to avoid deficiency problems.

Some of my readers have had trouble finding this vitamin in the proportions mentioned above. At the end of the book, under sources for various foods, supplements, and items of use, there is an address of a reputable company to which you may write for a supply of these vitamins. By all means, try and find the formula locally before you order by mail. It could be slightly cheaper to buy from a local source.

CHAPTER SEVEN

PEOPLE AND SITUATIONS
THAT KEEP YOU FAT

This chapter covers a number of situations that might or might not apply to you. They are educational in that you can build up some knowledge of the tactics of saboteurs, not to mention learning how to deal with these people. One of the hardest tasks that a dieter has is the survival in the food jungles that he or she must constantly go near in everyday living. A dieter is literally not safe anywhere, not even in church.

SEX AND WEIGHT LOSS

I am using the word sex as a generic term and am referring to the relationships between men and women that could affect how an obese person performs on a slimming program. A slimmer has to deal with the feelings of his or her spouse, other members of the opposite sex, and even persons of the same sex. A few case histories may illustrate some of the problems facing someone trying to get rid of unwanted pounds in a hostile environment.

Anne

This patient is a 43-year-old woman who is married to an alcoholic. She married him at age 15 to escape an alcoholic and sexually abusive father. Leon, her Prince Charming, soon became her alcoholic jailer. When first seen by me she weighed 250 pounds and had a number of medical problems, including hypertension. Her blood pressure was not helped much by the fact that she had four children, a house to keep clean, a job at a local garment factory, and a drunken husband who refused to work because of his "nerves." He was, however, able to drink and stayed at home all day doing that job.

Her own mother had died of the effects of hypertension and Anne was motivated enough to lose 47 pounds over the next five months. The hypertension improved, but her home life did not. She had to hide the fact that she was seeing us for her weight problems, but she could not hide the continuously shrinking figure and the need for constant alteration of her clothes.

She was met at the door each night after work with tirades from Leon about how she had been "stepping out" on him with another man. She was told that he would kill her if she left him. After a particularly bad beating, she finally left and is seeking a divorce as I write this.

There often seems to be a pairing of overweight women and alcoholic men. The basic insecurity usually found in these men leads them to seek out a fat wife. If she is not fat to begin with, he arranges the circumstances so that she becomes (and stays) obese. Efforts by these women to lose fat are met with ridicule, sabotage, and abuse, often of the physical variety.

This type of man (if we can call him that) is deathly afraid of losing his wife, usually because of his neglect or abuse of her over the years. He is unwilling to improve himself and feels any loss of weight by her is a threat. His sometimes deeply buried guilt, if he feels any at all, surfaces, and he projects his own feelings into what he perceives as her's. The long years of neglect on his part come home to him, and he realizes that she might find someone else if she is more attractive and slimmer than before.

The efforts by the husband to stop this weight reduction process are sometimes more than the abused wife can fight, and her husband wins again. Usually if the woman is made aware of the dynamics of her relationship with her alcoholic spouse, she can work through the problems and still regain her normal weight. In the process she may reassure him enough to keep from being abused, or she will get rid of the alcoholic millstone around her neck and assert her own independence and self-worth. Anne did the latter and by the time you read this she should be single.

Her husband has broken into her new home on three different occasions since she left him, but a rather stern female judge has assured him that if he harasses Anne again, the penalties will put him out of reach of his liquid refreshments for a long time to come. What this patient did was not easy, but at least she now has a chance for a better life and a healthier body.

Charlie

Charlie is a salesman and is gone most of each day on sales calls. He was a football player at one of the local universities 20 years ago and is still remembered as a star fullback by the alumni. His wife, Faye, married him not long after graduation but had been quite jealous of him during their courtship. She soon solved the problem of her football hero "hunk" by making him into a "hulk" instead.

Two decades of too much food, too little exercise, too much drinking, and an almost insane insistence by Faye that he clean his well-filled plate every meal produced a medical disaster for me to deal with. His 75 inches of height were still too short for his 320 pounds, and it became apparent that he was in Coronary Country. An extremely bad family history of arteriosclerotic heart disease made matters even worse. All of his brothers and his father, along with two paternal uncles, had died of heart disease before the age of 45, not a pleasant prognosis for my 41-year-old patient.

Faye seemed happy with Charlie. After all, he was home every night to eat the massive meals she prepared for him. A referral to my office produced no such happy feelings in our minds. Charlie was told of his imminent danger and advised of a number of risk-reduction steps I wished him to take. Efforts to get Faye to come in and receive instructions in how to help reduce his risks met with evasions, and finally, outright hostility on her part.

How dare I tell her how to cook for her family! She was a good wife and mother and did not appreciate some stranger telling her how to do things. It became clear that we would have to do things without Charlie's wife, and we started under this rather severe handicap. Charlie began a comprehensive program of combined dieting, behavior modification, and a long walk every night, instead of plopping down in front of the television with snacks prepared by Faye to keep him from being hungry between dinner and bedtime.

His weight loss was magnificent! He lost an average of four pounds each week and had lost over 80 pounds in five months. Then disaster hit Charlie. He had eaten an early breakfast each morning, usually prepared by him, instead of his late-sleeping wife. It was exactly as specified. Lunch was fortunately a simple matter of eating in the local Wendy's with judicious use of their salad bar and his own low-calorie dressing that he took with him. Dinner at home became the big problem for Charlie.

Fay kept on preparing the massive evening meals, in spite of his refusal to eat these impossibly fattening foods. As he approached 240 pounds, she became more and more abusive, often keeping him up all night with her screaming and tantrums. She began to follow him to work and to exhibit paranoid tendencies, accusing him of seeing other women during the day. The abuse finally wore Charlie down and he gave in to her.

He rapidly gained 30 of the pounds he had lost, much to the satisfaction of his jealous wife. It took a bout of chest pain and the need for a triple coronary artery bypass to convince Faye that she could have him fat and dead, or thin and perhaps with a chance to keep him around long enough to see his grandchildren. I finally persuaded her to go to a therapist and work out some of her anxieties about having a slimmer husband.

I am happy to report that Charlie now weighs slightly over 210 and is free of symptoms of coronary artery disease. Faye is now supportive of his efforts and realizes how narrowly she escaped being a relatively young widow.

Susan

Susan first came to me eight years ago with a number of problems besides her obesity. She was the widow of an Army major who had died in a helicopter crash. She and her teenage son lived with her parents. Both her mother, who had severe heart disease, and her father, an emphysema victim, were chronically ill and dependent on their only daughter.

What started as a temporary stay with them soon turned into an almost parasitic relationship. If she was five minutes late coming in from her secretarial job in the afternoon, she was bombarded with questions as to where she had been. Didn't she know how sick they both were? Didn't she know how much they needed her to help them? Any attempts to go out at night, even to church, were met with more nagging and questions.

Her one try at going out on a date during this eight year period was met with a "heart attack" performed by her mother. This almost Academy Award performance induced Susan to break her date, alienating a possible suitor and tying her even closer to her parents. Both her parents worked on her less-than-assertive nature to get their way.

All her money and most of her free time were drained from her life by these parental tyrants until their deaths about a year ago. Since then she has begun to live her own life a little more but is still timid about dating. Finally, for the first time since she started coming to me, I have been able to help her get a substantial amount of fat off. She is no longer verbally abused, nagged, or shamed into eating portions that would choke a field hand. She now does her own cooking.

Fear and selfishness on her parents' part kept her bound to them. The bonds were made of guilt, excess food she was bullied into eating, and a life style that did not encourage exercise or other recreation. All she needed was freedom in order to change her life and her figure. Her 65-inch-tall body that once carried over 235 pounds now weighs 127.

The Chubby Chaser

Ivan is a 30-year-old delicatessen owner who is successful and prosperous. His mother, a massively overweight woman, died when he was 18, and Ivan has never gotten over her loss. Because his mother was such a caring and loving woman, her weight never seemed to bother him or his father. For the past ten years he has run his delicatessen and has had a series of love affairs with women who are as fat or fatter than his mother.

While refusing to commit himself to marriage with any of these women, he has had a relatively active sex life with as many as six or seven of them at any one time. He is not in the least repelled by their collective adiposity. In fact, the more massive the woman, the greater his passion and desire for her. When not making love with them, he is cooking and serving each of them (one at a time, of course) as much food as she wants.

A few have slimmed down, hoping to perhaps catch this eligible bachelor, only to find themselves rejected for being too skinny. Ivan has an aberration known as "Chubby Chaser Syndrome." It is harmless, and I'm sure it provides attention and sex to some women who might otherwise be without either. Ivan is, in essence, looking for and finding a mother substitute. Marriage is out, since one might love one's mother but should not marry her.

A few frustrated Chubby Chasers wind up with a slim wife by mistake, but they soon correct this problem. A couple of pregnancies and a lot of food later, and she is fat enough to conform to this type of man's standards of beauty. Ivan and others like him are not as malicious as some mates mentioned earlier, but a Chubby Chaser will not help a woman in her quest for thinness if she is married to one or contemplating it.

THE MESSAGE

The message behind each of these true stories is that other people may have something to gain or lose, depending on how successful you are on a slimming program. Sometimes jealousy or insecurity is the motivating force. Sometimes there is not even a conscious effort to be a saboteur, but the results are the same. It pays for each patient to look at every personal contact he or she has with others during the day. Look for the supportive people and hold on to them. Also, look for the instances in which another person has overtly, or in a subtle way, been able to influence your eating or drinking behavior pattern.

Practice the Cognitive Restructuring (CR) exercises that are mentioned in the next chapter. Practice saying "NO" mentally many times in an expected or imagined situation. When the situation comes up, you are ready because you have already lived it a number of times in your mind and imagination.

You may have to break off contact with certain "friends" and relatives, either forever or for a long enough time for you to be strong and assertive enough to resist their efforts to feed you. Feeders may have obvious motivations, as well as deep-seated ones. Be suspicious of anyone offering you, a dieter, problem foods and beverages. Remember the old Freudian statement: "Just because you are paranoid doesn't mean that everyone isn't against you!"

The last group of items in this chapter are aimed at specific targets, the saboteurs who might try and wreck your diet. The Feeder section is a warning to beware those who, for their own reasons, are out to ruin your diet. The open letter to a spouse, parent, or friend of a patient is a plea for help that might give someone insight into his or her influence on a patient. The section "What is a Thief?" is another attack on those who might try to slow a person's weight loss down.

FEEDERS AND OTHER SABOTEURS

Any person who is even moderately successful in losing unwanted pounds will probably run into one or more of this type of person. If you are aware of the tactics that are used by feeders, your success will be much more likely and your life will be a lot simpler. I will give a few case histories in this chapter to illustrate just how deadly these saboteurs are. The destructive influences of a spouse of an obese patient are somewhat different in their patterns and will be covered in a separate section.

Obesity is a killer disease and one would think that no rational and compassionate person would attempt to stop an overweight person from losing. Such is not the case. Almost all of my patients have encountered this situation, some more than others. There are three basic types of feeders, each with a slightly different reason for being that way. Each of them will be covered in detail. I will be using feminine pronouns, but there are also male feeders and saboteurs too!

The Thin Feeder

All of us have seen situations where a thin woman seems to cultivate the friendship of a woman who is much heavier than she is. If the thin feeder is truly thin, the overweight woman makes her look even thinner. Someone who is 20 pounds over her desired weight will still look thin if compared to her friend who has 50 pounds to lose. If this obese friend begins to lose weight and starts to look more attractive, the relationship is threatened and the thinner of the two feels the competition, either real or imagined. The usual behavior of the thin feeder is to try and sabotage her friend and think up places to go where the supply of forbidden foods is abundant. If this fails to work, and it will fail where the dieter has been given a good orientation and warning about this phenomenon, the newly slim woman will find herself without this particular "friend."

Carol and Sally were friends and co-workers in an insurance office in Atlanta. Carol was slightly obese but had managed to never exceed 15 pounds over her ideal weight. Sally, a recent divorcee, was the mother of three small children and had gained 80 pounds over her desired weight of 120 pounds. She was friendly and a hard worker and made Carol seem almost anorexic in comparison. The two of them went to lunch each day and often shopped together as well. A physical in my office showed that Sally had elevated cholesterol and triglycerides, hypertension, and a symptomatic hiatal hernia.

The initial remedy for all of these problems was weight reduction using a fat-controlled diet. Eating out was forbidden, with only food prepared at home to be consumed at work. Fast foods and sweets were to be avoided. Sally now had to walk during her lunch hour and had no more time to eat and shop with Carol. She lost at a steady rate of eight pounds a month, reaching a weight of 160 in five months. She noticed that Carol began to bring in sweets to the office and also would conspicuously leave her a helping on her desk, even though she repeatedly asked her not to do so.

After two or three binges on sweets brought on by this subtle type of sabotage, she discussed this with me. A study of her food intake diaries showed that her office was the only place where she had dieting problems. The instigator in each case was Carol. We discussed the problem and decided to use the Parrot Technique (see the section on Dealing with Pests). The weight loss resumed at its old rate, and within another six months she was down to her desired weight and placed on a maintenance program.

Her blood pressure, blood fats, and hiatal hernia symptoms were all improved. She felt wonderful, except that she had to make new friends. Carol, her former close friend, and some of the other office workers had virtually ostracized her. They continued to try to get her to fatten up again by offering tempting food but refused to include her in their social activities. Fortunately, she was warned of this and had ignored their hostile acts. She had been made aware of the dynamics of feeder behavior and had accepted the situation. Sally now is in her second year of maintenance and has a lot of new and slimmer male and female friends. She has discovered how she was being used and refuses to be a victim any longer.

The Overweight Feeder

A lot of obese women do not like to be seen in public alone. This is particularly true if public eating is involved. If one overweight female is in an ice cream parlor eating a large sundae, it could make her self-conscious. If five obese ladies are together and eating the same thing, there seems to be a feeling of mutual support. They are eating buddies and help bolster each other's courage in violating their "diets" that they claim to sometimes follow.

If one of their number becomes a success at dieting and starts shedding pounds and inches, the others may attack with food and temptations involving obviously fattening foods and beverages. There may be remarks from them that the dieter is looking sick, looking wonderful, looking wrinkled, and other equally disparaging or discouraging comments. Whatever the statement, it is always followed by an invitation, a request, or even a virtual order to eat "just a little bit" of whatever is most fattening.

The overweight feeder is afraid of losing an "eating buddy" and is also certainly quite jealous. A shark or wolverine has more compassion than a feeder, as this next story will illustrate.

Elaine was a teacher at a local elementary school. Her initial weight on seeing me was 300 pounds. She had developed problems with her back that caused her extreme pain and disability. It was obvious to her orthopedist and to me that there was no choice but to get her weight down as quickly as possible. She was placed on a variant of the protein sparing modified fast and followed closely. Weight loss was a predictable four pounds a week, with no problems with electrolytes or hunger.

Elaine had previously been part of a group of six unmarried or divorced teachers who were all significantly overweight. One of the six, Hannah, had less fat to lose, but started at the same time as Elaine. By the time Elaine had lost the first 50 pounds, Hannah had dropped out in response to the pleas of the other four in the group. The usual method of sabotage was to place, unwanted and unrequested, a plate of sweets or concentrated calories of some other type in front of Hannah and Elaine. The feeder would then implore both of them to eat something, "since it was fixed just for you."

Elaine refused to be the victim of these food bullies, but Hannah was not able to assertively refuse and eventually got discouraged, resumed her old eating habits, and rapidly regained all of her weight, plus 15 pounds. The others in the group, now including Hannah again, began to make things unpleasant for Elaine. She was told that she was getting ugly and wrinkled and that she had really gotten "stuck up" since she lost that weight. In spite of her still needing to lose over a hundred pounds more, she was told that she didn't need to lose any more. Her temperament and disposition were attacked as being terrible, and other uncomplimentary things were said about her.

Elaine had been instructed early on about the tactics of feeders and was unmoved by all these increasingly disagreeable remarks. She continued to lose weight and got enough confidence in her own abilities to resume her post-graduate studies. Her increased self-esteem helped her overcome what could have been an overwhelming negative influence on her efforts. She is now principal of another school and has only a few more pounds to lose at the time this history is written. She has also found herself attractive enough and slim enough to date several eligible men. Unfortunately, her five former friends are still part of a coven of overeaters, none of whom have been able to break away from the others and get rid of their unwanted poundage.

The almost malignant influences of the thin feeder and the fat feeder are difficult to combat, but neither type is as deadly and as hard to fight as the next one.

The Grandparent Feeder

Again, I will refer to a grandmother figure when this type of feeder is discussed, but there are as many grandfathers in this category as there are female grandparents. This type of person may not actually be a grandparent and may not even be old, but the archetype is the granny figure with a plate of brownies or some other equally diet-destroying food.

"Now Sonnie (or Missie), you *know* that this little bit of food can't possibly hurt you. This diet business is silly. Besides, this couldn't be unhealthy. I made it with pure cream. You're not going to break your poor granny's heart and not have some. I made them just because I knew you were coming to see me." It would be almost a sin to refuse this kind of plea, particularly since you know that love motivated her, not jealousy or envy.

This type of feeder feels that love is shown best by feeding. Any attempt to reject the food offered is a rejection of the grandparent feeder's love, a difficult thing to spurn. Most dieters find that frequent telephone calls, instead of visits, to this type of feeder is the best way to maintain contact. The grandmother figure is hard to deal with in person. It is also impossible to convince her that you are right in losing your attractive baby fat, even if you are the parent of grown children yourself. Take my advice and love her from a distance. Give her your phone number, but not your address. She will mail you sweets and fattening foods otherwise.

All of these examples should make you more observant of your own surroundings. It would pay each person on a reducing diet to observe his or her environment during seven consecutive days. List everyone who even remotely offers you food or beverages during that time. List people who made you eat, even if they triggered you to eat through annoyance or some other emotion and didn't actually offer food.

Try and figure out the tactics of each one and see how his or her influence could be overcome. Work out your own methods of dealing with each one and practice these mentally before you actually encounter the person again. Use cognitive restructuring as I have illustrated it in the chapter following this one. Your life as a dieter and maintainer of a slim figure will be much less complicated, not to mention more pleasant and healthier.

AN OPEN LETTER TO THE SPOUSE (OR PARENT, OR FRIEND) OF MY PATIENT

You may think that this is a rather unconventional thing to do, appealing to someone close to a dieter for help, but certain things need to be said to you or all the dieter's efforts will possibly be for nothing and the dieter will fail. For this reason, please carefully read everything that follows. All the things mentioned in this letter do not apply in every case, but they are used as examples of things that could go wrong.

It is obvious that no one holds an overweight person down and makes him or her overeat. In 99 percent of the cases, the person who is overweight is that way because he eats more food than he burns. What is not so obvious is the effect that the environment has on the overweight individual. Numerous scientific experiments have pointed out, time and time again, that the surroundings and external influences on a fat person have more to do with his problem eating behavior than the internal cues of hunger have ever had.

A large majority of overweight persons never experience a true feeling of hunger or of satiety (lack of hunger) in the way that an individual of normal weight does. Certain experiments have shown that cues, such as elapsed time from the most recent meal, odors, sight of food (watching TV and eating), being in a certain location, and emotional upset will trigger massive food intake at times. These cues can make even the most compliant dieter vulnerable to problem eating impulses.

You may be asking yourself, "What does all this have to do with me? It is not my problem. He (or she) should be able to diet by will power alone! Why involve me at all? If she (or he) does not do well, the overeating is not my fault."

Nothing could be further from the truth. You are important, in fact, more important than most of the people in this dieter's life, or you would not be reading this now. If you are truly interested in helping the dieter, please take what is said here on faith for a while and see for yourself whether or not it is true. It may mean changing your own life style a bit, but the results will be worthwhile.

To begin with, never criticize the dieter for not dieting properly or for his or her eating habits. Ridicule, teasing, taunting, or other verbal abuse does not stop an undesirable behavior. It most likely will only make him or her want to eat more than before. You may have to bite your tongue to do so, but only comment on desirable eating behavior. If the patient is not breaking the diet, then comment on how good that behavior is. If a lapse does occur, and this will happen, the less said, the better. In the long run, positive reinforcement techniques work better for compliance to a diet plan. To repeat, even if you see something done incorrectly, please say nothing.

Since visual or olfactory (odor) cues are important in producing undesirable eating behavior, the dieter needs to "fat-proof" his or her dwelling. This means that all junk food that might be tempting must be cleaned out. For the rest of your family or social group, it might mean going out to get ice cream and refusing to eat it, or something equally tempting, in front of the dieter. To eat such goodies in front of someone on a diet is the height of cruelty.

Many families are used to eating together, but the dieter may decide not to eat with you if distress is caused by sitting and watching others eat. He or she may simply eat quickly and then get right up from the table after finishing, even if others have not yet stopped eating. Many dieters are pickers, and if such a person remains at the table, it will be difficult not to nibble at one thing or another. Please be understanding, and at a later date, when dieting efforts have been successful, normal table behavior may be resumed.

A dieter may have to stay away from problem places, such as pizza parlors, taco stands, spaghetti houses, hamburger stands, take-out fried chicken stores, doughnut parlors, and other equally tempting dens of obesity. Please do not bring this type of food home and tempt the dieter. The result is usually disastrous and is equivalent to tempting an alcoholic to go into a bar, or to bringing him or her a bottle of whiskey. No thinking and caring person would do that to an alcoholic, but lots of people will try to "feed" a dieter.

What this message boils down to is that the dieter is weak and does have some bad habits, but he or she is worth any and all efforts to help save him or her from the life-shortening effects of obesity. You and others may be inconvenienced a little, but surely you can tolerate these minor annoyances for a while.

About one of every hundred dieters is faced with open or hidden sadism, or mental illness, on the part of his or her spouse or a relative.

A certain type of person seems to feed on the misery of others, particularly of those who are overweight. One example is the husband who keeps his wife fat, usually because of insecurity or other related reasons. He feels secure because she is so obese that no one else would have her. When his wife tries to lose weight, such a man becomes anxious and tries to get her to go off the diet by tempting her, annoying her, or by otherwise sabotaging her efforts. As she gets closer to her lower weight goal, he becomes more and more anxious and will resort to physical abuse, verbal assaults, and as a last desperate effort, may cut off her funds so that she cannot continue her weight program. For those who stick it out and continue the diet program, there is sometimes divorce, usually coming on the heels of an increasing amount of verbal and physical abuse.

Not all victims are wives. Many are husbands of insecure wives, or children of insecure parents. Some men are victims of a bullying, feeding wife. These women try to get and keep what they want, a husband so fat and unattractive that no one else would want him.

In summary, you and others who have close contact with the dieter have more influence on him or her than you could ever realize. Without your total assistance and support, the dieter will more than likely fail. The attitude that "food is love" is widespread. The idea is still strong in many people that by giving food you show love, and by rejecting that food you also reject that love. You can, however, show love in ways not related to food. Try flowers and small, inedible (not made of chocolate) gifts to show affection and love. They work just as well and last a lot longer! Please let me know if I, as this person's therapist, can help you in your efforts to be supportive to my patient.

WHAT IS A THIEF?

There are many varieties of thieves in the world, but the most vicious of all are those who steal something of great personal value from another person. The thing stolen doesn't need to have resale value in order to make the crime of theft a serious one. Sometimes, the item that is stolen away from the owner is health, happiness, and self-respect.

The person who is trying to diet and lose unwanted fat moves through a jungle of food cues and temptation every day. In a large percentage of cases this person *must* lose the fat in order to prevent serious health problems, or to lessen the seriousness of an illness already existing. Fat loss will make the person better and healthier, both mentally and physically. Fat gain, or lack of fat loss, will perpetuate the problems that already exist in the patient's health situation.

With all these pressing needs you would think that nobody in his or her right mind would attempt to get a dieter to go off a weight loss program. It is both disappointing and a source of anger to me that someone would, indeed, try to sabotage another's plan of fat loss and self-improvement. Almost daily I am told by some luckless patient that he or she was literally bullied by some moron into eating or drinking something that was forbidden. At the time the dieter did not have the ability or the strength to resist but later was overcome by guilt and remorse while the culprit went happily off to seek another victim.

The purpose of this last section is to make you aware of this problem and to suggest some remedies. In the process it is hoped you will launder your mind of guilty thoughts and look closely at this type of saboteur. In a previous section of this chapter I called them Feeders, but they could also be called Thieves and Scoundrels.

Each month you put out a substantial amount of time and effort and money in order to purchase and earn your goal of a thinner and healthier body. This effort and money have a certain value to you. Anyone who would deliberately try and wreck your diet with "just a little bite of this," and with the admonition "Come on and try it, it won't hurt your diet," is stealing something of great value from you and should be treated like a Thief and Scoundrel.

Even if you dismiss these tempting words as the mouthings of a fool, you still are being put at risk and are in danger of going off your diet because of these sabotage efforts. Since only a fool or malicious busybody would try and wreck your diet program, you owe this person no courtesy or consideration. Treat him or her with the contempt he or she deserves and try to remove this person from your life if you can. If you can't totally avoid him or her, try to minimize your contacts and live your life and diet as you see fit. Become more assertive and firm in your answers if there is no way to escape him or her. You might even show the person these pages. Maybe this deliberately blunt and admittedly unpleasant group of comments will penetrate even this individual's thick skull!

CHAPTER EIGHT

COGNITIVE RESTRUCTURING IN SLIMMING

Cognitive restructuring (CR) refers to a process of changing a person's thinking and his or her responses to a particular situation. Cognitive literally refers to the thinking and reasoning processes. In the case of those trying to lose unwanted fat, the goal is to change fat thinking into slim thinking.

A lot of the effectiveness of CR is related to the practice sessions carried out by a slimmer or dieter. The particular conditions and situations are thought out, then a desirable and practical response by the slimmer is imagined and written down in an outline by the person attempting to modify his or her behavior. The consequences of each response are analyzed and a decision is made as to whether or not this response is a desirable one, producing desired results. It seems cumbersome and involved at first, but it is really a simple and effective process. For example:

SITUATION: You are out shopping with a friend and she suggests you both go to a restaurant where you know there is NOTHING much you can eat on your weight loss program. In the past, every time you have gone there, it has been a disaster and you pig out. There are other restaurants in the area that are kinder to slimmers. What do you do?

RESPONSE NUMBER ONE: Go along and try to survive at the problem restaurant.

RESPONSE NUMBER TWO: Tell your friend that you want to have lunch with her, but would rather go to _____ (a restaurant with a salad bar and less problematic foods).

After looking at these two possibilities, you obviously would pick number two. It is likely that you could make your friend upset or annoyed, but you can practice being persuasive to her many times in your mind before the actual situation might occur again. You have already responded to her in your mind so many times, making it more likely that you will active in an assertive manner. This is a good opportunity for you to find out if she is really your friend or just an acquaintance.

SITUATION: You are in a grocery store and have been shopping for your weekly food needs. You are exactly on your diet program and have been for some time. You are walking by a store food display and a salesperson tries to give you a taste sample of your favorite sweet (cookie, cake, candy, etc.). You see this favorite sweet and smell its aroma. You imagine how good it would taste and are sorely tempted. Your child (who should have been left at home) begins to beg, plead, and bully you into tasting the sample offered, not to mention buying some, too.

RESPONSE NUMBER ONE: Give in and eat the sample and feel guilty immediately. Begin to feel so guilty that you buy several packages of the sweet and go on a binge.

RESPONSE NUMBER TWO: You politely refuse and rapidly steer your cart to another aisle in the store, resolving to either (a) kill or maim your child at the first opportunity (remember, this is a mental exercise only), or (b) never bring him or her back to the store again, or (c) do both (a) and (b).

You can see that these responses also tell you what not to do, such as going to shop for groceries with your child. You won't be able to imagine all the situations that could affect you at one sitting, but your continuing experience as you slim will build your list of situations that could threaten your compliance to a diet. Here is one more and then there will be space for you to write some of your own.

SITUATION: You are at a family reunion with a lot of your aunts, grandparents, cousins, and other relatives. The table is literally groaning under the weight of some of your favorite foods, none of which is really permitted on your program yet. Some of these relatives know you have been losing fat and are pestering you to eat more. They tell you that you look bad and should not lose any more weight. They even try to shovel food on to your plate when you refuse to go get it yourself.

RESPONSE NUMBER ONE: Give in and hope you can get back on your program when you get away from these pests. Say nothing to them and don't try to fight their attempts to sabotage you. Feel so guilty later that you continue to binge and quit your diet program.

RESPONSE NUMBER TWO: Tell everybody to leave you alone. Get actually unpleasant with each of them, enough to alienate them for life. Leave early and plan to never attend one of these reunions again.

RESPONSE NUMBER THREE: Bring your own food, including lots of raw and lightly steamed vegetables. Quietly make sure that your plate is FULL of food, but your OWN food. Save up a lot of your daily food allotment for this meal with your relatives. The saving and the bringing of your allotted food requires planning, so make up your mind that this is necessary. Scout the food spread that your relatives have laid out on the table. Pick and choose a couple of items that conform to your slimming program. Go back several times, getting a small quantity of one item each time. Eat slowly and stay on your program during the

125

entire social function. In response to requests to eat something that was made "just for you," say that you will possibly do so later. Leave the reunion happier than you would have been because of your success at staying on your routine under pressure.

See? It's not that hard to mentally work things out. Now it's your turn to practice. On the next few pages are a few blank CR practice forms. Fill them out, or make new ones of your own. Good luck, both on your mental exercises and in the real thing.

SITUATION:

RESPONSE NUMBER ONE:

RESPONSE NUMBER TWO:

RESPONSE NUMBER THREE:

CONSEQUENCES OF MY CHOICE OF ACTION:

DUTCH DIET

SITUATION:

RESPONSE NUMBER ONE:

RESPONSE NUMBER TWO:

RESPONSE NUMBER THREE:

CONSEQUENCES:

SITUATION:

RESPONSE NUMBER ONE:

RESPONSE NUMBER TWO:

RESPONSE NUMBER THREE:

CONSEQUENCES:

CHAPTER NINE

HYPOGLYCEMIA, THE GREAT IMITATOR

I was eating lunch in a restaurant in a San Francisco hotel a few years ago, while attending a medical convention. The young waitress who took my order noticed a medical article reprint I was reading and wanted to know if I was a doctor. I replied that I was, and that my interests were mostly confined to nutrition and the treatment of the overweight patient. This, I found out, is something you should never mention to certain people, in this case a tall, blond hysteric.

She told me that she was from Philadelphia and had moved away a few years ago. She never seemed to keep a job, usually leaving each one after a month or so. Being a waitress was easier, because if she didn't like one job there was always an opening somewhere else.

Her symptoms read like a textbook presentation of the hysteric patient. The expressions she used were repetitive and included "Really!" and "Like WOW!" and "You know," not to mention "Heavy" and others. She was plagued by symptoms that sounded, at a tableside consultation, to be related to depression and hysteria.

She said, "You know, I'm going to like this really cool doctor here in town. He told me that like, all my troubles are related to low blood sugar. I get these injections in the veins three times a week. It's, like I mean, something to do with the adrenal glands. I'm feeling great, and like WOW, I really get off on these shots. Really! The only bad thing is that I can't eat like, any refined sugar, white flour, or processed foods. I also can't drink any more and it's, like a drag, you know."

She had, indeed, improved on the treatment for her "hypoglycemia." Part of it could have been a more nutritious diet, but this might have been learned by her at a lower cost than the $30.00 she paid for visits to her doctor three times a week. Part of it might have been her cutting down on her alcohol consumption and getting more rest. I imagine that the major part was being able to place the majority of the blame for her symptoms on a clearly defined diagnosis (which was probably in error, as you shall see) that could allow her to ignore personality problems that also needed attention and help.

The hypoglycemia mills that flourished in the past few decades have been fueled by the numerous books and lectures by "authorities" on the subject. Go into any health food store today and read the pamphlets and paperbacks that are sold and given away there. Want to invest a few hundred dollars quickly? If so, just ask the proprietor or clerk a simple question. Such as, what would he or she recommend for your minimal vitamin and mineral supplement intake?

Whether or not these vitamins and minerals really do anything or not is a question we won't address here, but most physicians are of the opinion that these vitamins and minerals are overused. Each of the major vitamins and minerals is covered in the chapter on the subject, so I won't belabor it here, but these necessary substances are often taken for reasons that have their basis in anecdotal accounts only.

This is not to suggest that health food stores are cynical and mercenary in their zeal to sell these items. It has been my experience that most people in the health food industry are sincere in their beliefs, but perhaps flawed in their logic, about certain remedies they prescribe. Their pushing of hypoglycemia as a possibility is done as a result of their own experience. They have learned that a certain food or substance, when consumed, makes them feel ill, and not having it does not make them feel bad.

The medical literature is full of articles that attempt to explain and counter claims made by these "mills" that process the anxious and fatigued patients with injections instead of counseling to help with their symptoms and problems. What is particularly bad about the spurious treatment of a spurious disease is that many patients with real medical or psychological illness delay treatment for their actual problems because of the incorrect diagnosis of hypoglycemia.

Certain physicians and lay authors have influenced literally millions of people to look for their troubles inside a sugar dish, within a sweet confection, or at the bottom of a bottle of alcoholic beverage. It is true that usually it pays to avoid sugar, alcohol, or excess caffeine, but it might not be for the reasons given by these "experts."

The truth is that this problem is over-diagnosed by many lay and medical persons. The diagnosis gives both the "treater" and the treated a sense of security. Something IS wrong with him or her. It isn't "just in the mind." The person with these symptoms isn't "crazy or neurotic." There is something to treat. The placebo effect of dieting, getting good food, avoiding certain foods and beverages, stopping smoking, and perhaps increasing activity does tend to make the person feel better. Who is to say that these measures wouldn't help anyone?

The only harm might be in delaying treatment for some systemic disease that should have been diagnosed by a thorough medical evaluation, instead of a superficial look, or no look at the patient at all. Competent authorities have attacked the standards by which some patients are being diagnosed. One group of researchers found that about one out of 40 healthy asymptomatic patients had a glucose level that dropped below 39 mg/dl during a test.

Some who have studied hypoglycemia use what is known as the hypoglycemia index. It relates to the actual rate of drop in the blood glucose levels for the 90 minutes prior to the reaching of the nadir, or lowest level. It has not turned out to be clinically useful and does not seem to correlate with the symptoms exhibited by those tested.

Some doctors have shown in their studies that certain patients do have clinical symptoms of hypoglycemia following a glucose meal, but not after placebo testing was done using a non-caloric sweetened liquid. They diagnosed symptomatic hypoglycemia if hunger, rapid heart beat, perspiration, or numbness around the mouth were noted. These adrenalin-like responses are common in true hypoglycemia but can be seen in other states as well.

One authority calls some patients non-hypoglycemic, with the criteria being no symptoms or chemical evidence of true hypoglycemia. These were patients diagnosed as hypoglycemics by medical and non-medical "doctors" prior to their testing by his team. A substantial number of patients in their study showed undiagnosed somatic illness, including functional bowel syndrome, hypertension, ophthalmic migraine, pyelonephritis, tension headaches, and a heart condition known as idiopathic hypertrophic subaortic stenosis.

There was a lot of depression that was undiagnosed, or diagnosed and rejected by the patient, but still clinically significant depression. The phenomenon of denial is often present in a depressed person, causing them to turn to a clinical diagnosis, such as hypoglycemia, rather than face and remedy his or her real problem.

A large number of patients who seek the diagnosis of hypoglycemia are somatizers. Their symptoms make up an internist's nightmares, with fatigue, hyperventilation, "gland trouble," sleepiness during the day and insomnia at night, sexual problems of frigidity or impotence, weakness, tremor, voracious appetite,

panic reactions, and other equally vague but sometimes important clues to real systemic disease states. These somatizers also
grasp at the diagnosis of hypoglycemia as an "answer."

The somatizers will often exhibit classical symptoms of
hypoglycemia that they have memorized from lay books, even
when given nothing but non-caloric beverages. They will also
exhibit no symptoms when given glucose in capsules that hide
the sweet taste. There seem to be no definite norms for diagnosis of hypoglycemia. The fault may lie in what is given the
patient as a challenge meal. Many authors feel that the present
glucose tolerance test, using glucose beverage, is too artificial in
its makeup, producing artificial disease states. One medical
researcher and his associates in their 1981 article did note that
some of their patients did have symptoms following glucose
loading, in the absence of chemical hypoglycemia or elevated
plasma cortisol levels.

I have personally seen what I call pseudo-hypoglycemia
(PHG) in a number of patients who have no laboratory evidence
to back up the diagnosis. Even when the taste of glucose is
hidden from them by the use of capsules, they exhibit many of
the classical symptoms of hypoglycemia. Placebo capsules or
non-caloric beverages do not show this same symptom complex.

The health food industry and a lot of people in the nutrition
industry have labeled sugar a poison, particularly "white sugar."
I have found no basis in fact for their claims. My objection to
sugar lies in the over 128 pounds of empty calories in sugar
consumed every year by every person in this country. These are
often true empty calories but are harmless if caloric restriction
or the medical condition does not merit cutting down on sugar
intake. In the field of obesity treatment that amounts to a lot of
calories taken in every week, the absence of which would help
greatly in a patient's weight loss efforts.

Where PHG exists, or where there is a need for caloric
restriction for obesity or diabetes, I recommend initially a severe
restriction in sugar intake. Alternately, reasonable amounts of
fructose, sorbitol, mannitol, xylitol, saccharin, or aspartame

(Equal, Nutrasweet) could be used. Precautions in their individual use should be observed and their utilization reviewed with the physician prior to any extensive inclusion in a patient's diet.

The Malsovit bread used with this Dutch Diet is the ideal preventative measure for hypoglycemia or pseudohypoglycemia. In the bread is a complete protein and a slowly-absorbed source of carbohydrate that should not cause a rebound hunger within a few hours. I have personally experienced the long-lasting hunger-sparing effects of this product and recommend it highly.

In summary, hypoglycemia is a real entity. Fasting hypoglycemia can be a real herald of significant systemic disease. Postprandial (after meal) hypoglycemia, or reactive hypoglycemia is overdiagnosed, but is sometimes a real condition. Pseudohypoglycemia, as I call it, is also a real condition that responds to intelligent counseling and dietary management but without the expensive adrenal cortex extract injections that were formerly used. Physicians should make sure that all possible other sources for "hypoglycemic" symptoms are ruled out prior to assigning the patient to what, admittedly, may be a harmless and sometimes efficacious placebo diet involving avoidance, rather than active treatment.

Depression, in particular, should be watched for in all overweight patients. It is perhaps the most common diagnosis I make after evaluating chronically obese and frustrated patients. In my instruction classes for doctors, I tell them that the patient sitting across from each of them is not just a fat man or woman. He or she is a person with feelings and deserves their full attention, whether or not he or she is hysteric, depressed, fearful and acting out in an obnoxious way, or just plain scared at the prospect of being ill and disabled.

Doctor William Osler supposedly said, "Listen to the patient and he or she will tell you what is wrong." Let us hope that I and my colleagues never forget to talk to and listen to our patients when they come to us for help.

CHAPTER TEN

EXERCISE ROUTINES USEFUL FOR SLIMMERS

Exercise, or increased physical activity, is one of the three cornerstones of slimming. The other two important things are decreased caloric intake (of absorbable food) and changing the way a person deals with his or her environment. This rather short chapter will deal with exercise, but you will also read about its use in slimming in other places in *The Dutch Diet* book.

WALKING

Walking is one of the best forms of exercise for a slimmer. It is available to almost anyone, provided there is a safe place to walk. In our modern society we have to worry about traffic hazards, dangerous animals (both two-footed and four-footed), temperature extremes, uneven ground that might cause us to slip or fall, and the tendency to do too much at too rapid a pace.

The key word in walking for slimming is *patience*! Don't try to be too ambitious and do too much the first few days. The same defect in reasoning that makes an overweight person try to slim too strenuously is a problem here as well. Be realistic about what you can do to start with. If you are used to walking a half mile a day, then start with that and build up. If you haven't walked over a hundred yards at a time, start with that.

One of my heaviest patients is Herbert. He is 75 inches tall and initially came to me weighing over 660 pounds. His first walk was less than 100 yards. The next day he walked 150 yards and the next, 200. These round trips increased by 50 yards daily until he was walking over four miles a day. He is much thinner now, with a heart and lung capacity he didn't have when he started.

Each person has to realistically set an initial goal and try to meet it. The reasonably healthy person should try a *stroll* for the first few times for about 20 minutes. The pace may then be increased until it is relatively rapid and there is a feeling of exertion after the exercise period. After this goal is reached, the length of time and the distance may be gradually increased until a reasonable daily exercise routine is achieved.

To borrow from the "other" and more famous Doctor (Ken) Cooper, you must have some sort of training effect and use an aerobic type of exercise in order to achieve maximum results. The aerobic exercises that I favor are walking, swimming, running, use of the minitrampoline (rebounder), the Fitness Master exercise apparatus, and the stationary bicycle. I will cover each of these in some detail, but there are multitudes of books on each of these that cover it much better.

Sitting in a sauna, steam room, or whirlpool bath will make you feel good and make you sweat, but it doesn't get rid of anything but salt and water. Neither does sitting or leaning against a bunch of rollers at the spa. Massage also feels good but doesn't get rid of those excess pounds. Enjoy these things after exercise, but don't get a false sense of security from them.

You also shouldn't think you are "exercising" when you lift weights, whether with barbells and dumbbells, or with Nautilus-type equipment. It is true that you tone up, but this type of exercise is anaerobic and has no training effect on the heart. It is something that is nice to do if you need toning, but it isn't all you have to do.

Getting back to the subject of walking, this is as close as any exercise to being perfect for dieters in the beginning of their exercise routine. As the body's capacity increases, some dieters may want to jog or run. Please resist the temptation to do this until you get a good course of instruction from a knowledgeable runner. Many stores that sell runners' equipment also provide orientation and counseling on proper ways to warm up, to run, and to cool down afterwards. Take advantage of this knowledge, which usually comes at a minimal cost to you.

The cost in sprained or torn muscles and ligaments is far higher than a few extra dollars spent on proper shoes and instruction. There are also a large number of running books. Get your instructor's recommendations as to which ones might suit your needs better. If you are a man over 35, or a woman over 40, get an approval from your doctor before doing any strenuous exercise. Most physicians are able to either do a cardiac stress test on you or refer you to someone who can. This has been a life saver for a number of people who had what is called "silent heart disease" and who would have possibly harmed themselves by doing the wrong kind of exercise for their medical condition. Even doctors hurt themselves by running, as recently shown by the tragic death of Dr. Fixx.

With that warning out of the way, let me hasten to add that many heart consultants start their post-coronary patients on a specially tailored exercise program that includes walking. This is done very early following the heart attack or detection of an impending heart condition (angina pectoris). These patients usually receive great benefits from this. If you already have had a heart attack or onset of angina pectoris, you can still work an exercise program into your slimming regimen as long as your personal physician participates actively with you in your management.

When inclement weather prevents you from walking outside, consider a local enclosed shopping mall. If you are fortunate enough to have one of these handy, use it during rainy or excessively hot or cold days. If this is not feasible you might consider the next item, the rebounder.

THE MINITRAMPOLINE, OR REBOUNDER

A few years ago, I first encountered one of these devices at a meeting of the American Society of Bariatric (medical management of slimming) Physicians. I didn't even give the man who was selling them the courtesy of trying it out. In fact, I almost laughed in his face. What was such a ridiculous looking device doing at a weight control convention? I was so annoyed that I almost complained to the convention manager about letting such rubbish onto the exhibit floor.

Last year I changed my mind. After I had read a number of papers on the use of the rebounder and how the training effect was, indeed, a real factor in its use, I got two of them. One went into my office to use in showing patients how to use it correctly, and one went home with me. I have been able to demonstrate a definite training effect for patients who are relatively inactive and who want to tone up and increase their cardiac reserve. It does both of these things, and it does it indoors.

I would like to discuss how the rebounder is used and then what this means in terms of the body's response to this exercise. There are three basic things that the rebounder does when it is used properly.

The first activity on a rebounder is just bouncing up and down. All of us have probably been on a larger trampoline at one time or another. The effect is less on the rebounder, but the first effect, GRAVITY MASSAGE, is a real one. At the top of our bounce we are traveling upward and slow down. Just as we stop our upward movement and before we begin to fall toward the rebounder surface, we weigh slightly less than normal. We have all experienced this going up on a high speed elevator that decelerates as it takes us to a higher floor. As we fall down to the mat surface and decelerate again, there is another time when we stop movement temporarily. As our body hits the mat and depresses it, before we start the next upward bounce, we weigh slightly more.

When a person is bouncing up and down on a rebounder, and is doing so at an effective rate and with a significant amount of effort, an interesting thing takes place. Our changing back and forth, from weighing less at the top of the bounce and more at the bottom, produces a work effect on every muscle in the body. Each muscle works against gravity all the time, even the tiny muscles in the face and neck. If there is constantly changing gravity force, the muscles will, over a period of time, tone up and tighten up. This so-called gravity massage has an effect on some people that is close to amazing.

One of the most striking examples of this is Bertha (not her real name). Bertha is in her mid-fifties and had had a weight problem for a long time. She went into the business of selling rebounders and related exercise equipment, but primarily was in the accounting and paperwork end of the operation. She began to work on the rebounder every day and, over a month's time, worked up to 20 minutes of vigorous exercise twice a day. She followed a slimming program and was encouraged to see that the pounds fell off at a rate of two or three a week.

An unexpected bonus was the lack of loose skin over her body as she burned off the 50 or so excess pounds she needed to lose. Before, she had found that weight loss was accompanied by loose skin over her face, neck, abdomen, legs, and buttocks. This just wasn't the case when she combined the use of a rebounder with dieting.

Bertha is now a thin, healthy woman. She resembles a woman in her thirties, both in skin tone and in lack of wrinkles. Her rebounder has given her what I have called a medical face lift. If I hadn't watched the process over many months, I wouldn't have believed it myself. The rebounder may not give you as spectacular a result, but it certainly wouldn't hurt to try it.

The second thing a rebounder can do for you is to increase your exercise tolerance through its aerobic effect. It is possible to actually measure oxygen consumption in a laboratory, as well as the increase in heart rate while subjects are tested on the rebounder. Simply bouncing up and down will increase both of these. The training effect produced by bouncing and jogging in place will benefit almost everyone except a conditioned athlete. Highly trained people will not derive as much benefit from the rebounder as someone who isn't trained at all. This is not a problem since most of the people who want to lose weight are out of shape anyhow.

I usually encourage patients to go slowly. Stand on the rebounder surface and lightly bounce on it until you get used to it. Then bounce more vigorously. The same thing applies to someone who wants to run in place. Start slowly until you get your "sea legs" on the rebounder.

After you are comfortable with the bouncing effect, you can begin your exercise routine. I usually recommend running shoes and loose clothing that you might wear outside the house while running. Get yourself a disco record or something with a fairly constant beat to it. Also, try to find a large clock that has a second hand and put it in close view.

Start with about a minute of simple bouncing on the rebounder. Then run in place for a minute at about 120 steps a minute or better. Bounce on the rebounder for another minute and stop for the day. Don't try to do more than that on the first day. Add 30 to 60 seconds of running in place a day until you are at 20 minutes, then go to twice a day if possible. The warm-up rebounding should be gradually increased until you are bouncing three or four minutes before and after each running period.

There are a number of books about rebounding. Take some of them with a grain of salt. There is a lot of valuable information about using the rebounder for exercise. There is also a lot of misinformation that claims the rebounder is good for everything from cancer to ingrown toenails. Don't you believe it! It is a great tool for toning and conditioning the body, but that's all that it does. The average good quality rebounder can be purchased for a reasonable sum and is well worth its cost. If you don't yet have them in your area, write my publisher for further information as to where they can be purchased.

The third thing that a rebounder does is to protect your ankles, knees, hips, and other structures from the injury they could sustain while running on a hard surface. To illustrate my point, go to a place that sells rebounders and ask to try one out. Run in place on the floor for a few steps. Then, run in place on a rebounder. Lastly, run in place on the floor again. Do you feel the difference? It is amazing how few injuries occur on a rebounder as compared to those found in runners and even walkers. It can complement a walking program as an inclement weather alternative, or it can be the sole means of obtaining a good aerobic exercise pattern.

PADDLE AWAY YOUR POUNDS!

Not all patients can jog, walk briskly, rebound, or play racquetball. For them I recommend another excellent aerobic method of burning up excess calories and keeping the body muscles firmed up. Swimming is not always a possibility, but it is one that should be considered for many reasons.

When done properly for at least 25 to 30 minutes at a time, swimming is quite effective in producing a loss of calories. At first, it isn't necessary to swim laps to produce a training effect. Simple paddling around in the water will do a lot toward building stamina. It should be pointed out that standing in the water has a minimal effect but is not the ideal situation.

I instruct my patients who wish to use swimming as all or part of their exercise program to keep their swimming up for at least the 25 to 30 minutes mentioned above to begin with. At no time while in the pool can a patient touch the bottom with the feet, or the rails at the sides with the hands. There must be a constant and unrelenting effort to keep afloat by using the hands and feet. This paddling can burn up a tremendous amount of energy over a period of time and begins to strengthen the muscles for later, more vigorous swimming.

There is a second benefit of being mostly submerged in cool water—the heat lost from the body into the water. The amount of heat lost is dependent on the body temperature, the water temperature, and the surface area of the body that is exposed to the cool water. Heat, or calories, are lost in this way in a quite respectable amount. The greater the difference between body temperature and water temperature, the greater the amount of heat lost.

These calories lost into the pool water don't have to be burned by the body in muscular activity. This is an advantage to the dieter and helps accelerate the weight loss by this process. The opposite is true when a patient gets into a hot tub, sauna, or steam bath.

If it were possible, and if patients wouldn't get pneumonia in the process, sitting in a bath of cold water or inside a walk-in freezer locker for the same time they are baking in a sauna would get rid of more excess calories. Being in a hot environment doesn't mean you will gain weight, but it means there is little heat (calories) lost from the body in comparison to being in a cool or cold climate or environment.

If you decide to swim, make sure you are where there are adequate safety features, including a lifeguard or other capable person to watch you. NEVER SWIM ALONE!

Recently there have been a number of books written on aerobics performed while in a swimming pool. This can be a valid and useful exercise for those unable or unwilling to do these exercises under normal gravity conditions. The water supports a good part of your body while you are exercising, but the aerobic effect can still be felt.

One of the best books on water exercise has recently gone into its second edition. *HydroRobics* (aerobics in water) was written by Joseph A. Krasevec and Diane C. Grimes. It covers HydroRobics in general, plus exercises for the lower, middle, and upper body. There are enough illustrations and explanations for the average person to understand each exercise. I would recommend it highly to anyone interested in this form of exercise, particularly those with ankle, leg, knee, or hip injury, or those with back problems. It can be ordered by sending $9.95 plus $1.00 for bookrate postage to

HydroRobics Unlimited
P.O. Box 1106
Atlanta, GA 30301

Make checks payable to HYDROROBICS UNLIMITED

THE FITNESS MASTER

One of the most strenuous things I have ever attempted is cross-country skiing. The rhythmic motion of the legs and arms produced an aerobic exercise unlike anything else I have ever experienced. If I lived in Minnesota or Colorado, this would be one of my favorite activities.

Since I live in Georgia, there is little chance of snow skiing for me, but I found something almost as good. Something I can do indoors and do all year long. I acquired a Fitness Master aerobic conditioner and am well-pleased with it. It is light enough to carry with me in my car when I am away for several days. It is small enough to fit underneath my bed or to stand up in my closet. The Sierra unit that Fitness Master sent me is also well within the budgets of most of my readers. In short, it could turn out to be the perfect aerobic exerciser for me.

I have had two other experiences with similar, but not equal, machines. The mail order unit that was sold for less than $50.00 turned out to be totally inadequate and an actual joke as far as its poor construction and actions. I put it together out of curiosity and then gave it away. It wasn't even worth sending back, no matter how good the two models looked who were using it on television commercials.

The other unit was more substantial but mechanically inferior to the Sierra unit by Fitness Master. I didn't order it but saw it at a friend's house. He was moderately satisfied with the unit until he had tried out my Sierra. My unit had poles, rather than a system of pulleys. It was closer to my own experience with cross-country skiing and a lot easier to learn to use.

I particularly liked the informative guidelines for its use that the Fitness Master people sent with the Sierra. For information on this type of unit you can call them at 1-800-328-8995. Make your own decision after looking at the quality and prices of brands X and Y and comparing them to Fitness Master.

THE STATIONARY BICYCLE

Walking is the best of all the forms of aerobic exercise for slimmers, but sometimes there is no way for you to walk outside. The stationary bike is a reasonable alternative and can be placed in your home for a relatively small amount of money.

Regardless of the type of bike you purchase, it should be stable and sturdy, have a time, a speedometer, a mileage indicator, and a means of increasing the amount of resistance or tension present as you increase your exercise tolerance. Several of my patients have purchased their bikes at bargain prices by watching the want/sell ads in the local papers, reading their neighborhood shoppers, or putting a note on the bulletin board at work.

When you buy a bike, put it in front of your TV and "earn" your television programs by riding while watching. Keep the tension rather low and keep your speed constant at about 15 miles per hour to start with. The only thing that should change initially is the amount of time you spend riding. Start with about two minutes of riding and increase by 15 to 30 seconds a day until you are riding 20 to 30 minutes a day without stopping. Once you reach that level, you might want to ride two or three sessions a day for 20 minutes each exercise period. In the beginning it is best if you ride so that you can see a clock with a sweep second hand for more accurate timing. The secret is to *gradually* increase the workload so that your conditioning is smoother and more effective. This is a form of exercise that you can do every day of the year, rain or shine, day or night, in the privacy of your home. Plus, it works!

For a first-class exercise bicycle, the Schwinn Air-Dyne is my pick. The best isn't always the cheapest, however. The advantage of a Schwinn stationary bike of any type is that you usually have a Schwinn dealer near you and can take it to him, instead of having to ship it off to a factory service center. The price of around $600 is not out of line for the product.

The aerobic exercises mentioned in this chapter are not the only ones available, but they illustrate how flexible we can be in our choice of physical activity programs that are also aerobic. I would like for you to note how long it takes to burn 100 calories of energy in various activities.

ACTIVITY	TIME NEEDED TO BURN 100 CALORIES
Watching television	78 minutes
Walking, normal speed	19 minutes
Active bike riding	12 minutes
Active swimming	9 minutes
Active rebounding with running	9 minutes
Running	5 minutes

The above number of calories can be found in a large apple or two pats of butter. The calories may seem insignificant, but they add up. Alteration of the set point in slimming, another effect of exercise, is also quite important as I point out in another part of this book.

CHAPTER ELEVEN

GETTING IN TOUCH WITH YOUR BODY SIGNALS

This chapter is about what hunger is, and what it is not. You are reading this now because you have a problem with your eating. For many of you the thought of even a small level of deprivation of food is frightening. I understand this all too well. I was a fat medical student who became a fatter house officer, and later an even fatter physician. My top weight was slightly over 240 pounds in 1967, in spite of repeated attempts to diet and lose the excess pounds that I knew were shortening my life.

By the end of that year I had reached a goal of 180 and resolved never again to let my obesity and my "fat thinking" get the best of me. Such was not the case. I had lost on sheer nerve and fear of dying at too early an age. I had not really changed my thought patterns, as I will illustrate by the following true story.

I was in Charlotte, North Carolina, on a business trip. My plane was to leave there at about 7:00 P.M., but the Atlanta airport was fogged in and all incoming traffic was diverted. The airline provided a direct bus for the passengers trying to get to Atlanta, and I decided to take their offer and travel the four hours by bus instead of waiting to fly out of Charlotte the next morning. There was not time to get a proper dinner at the Charlotte airport, and I did not realize that the airline had provided a lunchbox for each passenger.

Something in me seemed to panic. I had to get something to eat! I would be out of reach of food for hours and I hadn't had any supper. The child in all of us came out in me. The next thing I knew I was standing in the line to get on the bus with four sandwiches, two cartons of milk, several packs of crackers, and a candy bar. Logic should have told me that any adult can delay eating for as much as an entire day without suffering any harmful effects. Four or five hours' delay in getting my evening meal would not have hurt me, but the fear of deprivation was still rooted deeply within my mind.

I look back on that episode as my first awakening to my real problem. I was still thinking like a fat man, in spite of my newly found slimness. It is funny now, but it was not so pleasant at the time. As you might guess, I survived the trip to Atlanta on the bus. I resolved then to take a good look inside my own mind and see how the flaws in my thinking processes affected me in everyday life. The information I gained from taking that look, plus the hints that I will be quoting in this and other chapters, should help you to see your own self a little more clearly. Self-knowledge is a powerful tool when used wisely.

Let's start with a simple statement that you may dispute but that has been proven to be true by some of the best medical and psychological researchers in the world. ***Most people with a weight problem never really feel true hunger or lack of hunger.*** Let me try to explain that rather surprising statement.

In numbers of well-controlled studies it has been shown that thin patients who were tested seemed to eat only when hungry. These slimmer people ate when hungry and refused to eat when hunger was not present. Their internal controls seemed to rule them, as opposed to external cues and influences. You can probably bear this out from your own observations of your more fortunate, and thinner, friends and acquaintances. You have observed them eating far more than you, with a lot of those foods being things you would not dare eat when trying to lose fat. They do all these seemingly fattening acts but stay thin.

A thin man or woman may choose to eat chocolate ice cream for lunch and nothing else. He or she may order the most fattening thing on the menu while you eat lettuce and cottage cheese. These fortunate people are governed by an internal control system that lets them eat what they want, when they want it, and how much they want. The difference between them and us (I still think somewhat like a fat man) is that they may only eat two or three bites of ice cream or pastry, then push the rest away uneaten.

You and I have trouble doing that. I make that assumption because almost all of us who are fat, or were fat, are like this. Your eating control is based mostly on external cues, or spurious and false internal cues. We will discuss some of these cues and how they affect you. We will also attempt to show you how they can be modified through education and by means of changing your environment or your response to it.

In the remainder of this chapter we will cover how you can change your entire life style over a period of several months. Gradual change is usually better than too rapid an alteration in your patterns of living. This section is one of the most important ones in your book. Knowing what to eat is a significant skill to learn, as is walking or exercising daily, but neither of the latter things is such a primary factor in your success. Thin thinking produces thin bodies, while fat thinking keeps you fat.

We have studied overweight men and women for years in an attempt to see why they are fat. This produced interesting studies and thousands of pages of data, but no answers. We only really made progress when we studied those who were thin without dieting. Duplicating what they do should produce the same degree of thinness for those of us who are less fortunate. It should work, and it has worked in my practice for the past 20 years or so.

Before we get into the actual mechanics of how to think differently, it is a good idea to deal with the so-called hunger that many of us experience. Like most physicians in private practice, I get bombarded with requests for "something to kill my appetite" by a lot of patients. A prescription for an anorectic agent may or may not produce sustained weight and fat loss. It usually doesn't over a period of time. The weight returns and the patient asks for "something stronger" to help with dealing with the demands of a weight loss program.

It is true that anorectic or "diet pills" can partially control true hunger in a patient. The problem is that what drives the person with a weight problem to eat will usually have nothing at all to do with hunger. The internal cues, that are somewhat blunted by medication, are not the problem anyhow. We are, therefore, attacking the problem from the wrong direction. Let's look at some of the "hungers" that often plague a patient and ruin a diet program.

When a patient comes to me with a complaint of the medication being too weak, or requesting medication because of what he or she perceives as hunger, I ask them to go through certain questions and look internally while doing so. The next paragraph lists some of the questions that are asked.

Are you really hungry? How do you know it is hunger? Where do you feel the hunger? How long was it between the time you finished a meal and when you felt hungry? Was it less than two hours? (If so the food is still in process of digestion and is being absorbed into the blood stream even as the "hunger" is being felt.) Do you feel any burning, emptiness, growling, spasm, or other uncomfortable feeling in the stomach area? What makes you think it is hunger instead of the normal contractions of the stomach that follow a few hours after a meal?

Most patients with these hunger pangs will find that a dose of antacid or a non-caloric liquid will usually quiet things down. Instead of a snack that could contain as much as 300 or more calories, the antacid will often abort the discomfort without the penalties of unwanted and unneeded food.

Another problem with "hunger" lies in the presence or absence of problem foods in the patient's daily surroundings. I have often gone for long periods of time without wanting problem foods until I was exposed to one or another of my own weaknesses in the snack category. As long as there were no Oreo cookies near me, I might think about them but would not go out of my way to have any. When they were brought into my home, or into my office, or near me at a relative's home, I was defenseless. Initially, if with other people, I would eat two or three. If I were alone, the entire package might be consumed during an evening.

In other parts of this book, techniques of behavior modification are discussed. Some of these ideas are repeated, but it is a good idea to mention some of them as they apply to the drive to eat. Whether you call this drive appetite or hunger doesn't matter for now. What is important is to get in touch with your body and mind and ask both of them every time you are about to purchase, accept, or eat something, if the food is really necessary to fuel your body or if you are eating and drinking it for other reasons.

Emotions and feelings can trigger inappropriate eating, even when a meal has just been eaten and there is no valid reason to eat. We tend to try and bury anger, sadness, depression, boredom, frustration, and other strong feelings under a mountain of foodstuffs. We return almost to infancy, to the thumb in the mouth, the full stomach (along with real or symbolic burping afterwards), the warm and comfortable feeling of oblivion, and the feeling of being loved that comes with being "full" again.

The empty feeling that a lot of problem eaters have may come from excess acid, or it may be more of a psychological emptiness than a real one. I usually remind my patients that the stomach is *supposed* to be empty most of the time. It is a receptacle and mixing station for foods, not the center of the universe.

I have my patients go through a drill that initially frightens them but later will give them a certain degree of confidence. They are told to eat a good lunch but to eat no evening meal or snacks after noon on a certain day. Each patient may have all the water and non-caloric beverages that are desired, but absolutely no food (not even lettuce) is allowed. Each person must look at the feelings experienced as an exercise in control. The questions about location, type, and degree of hunger are asked and answers are sought. I give each person some samples of liquid antacid to carry around, so that each one can experience the effect of putting something to neutralize acid into the stomach.

I have had people absolutely refuse to go without eating for even that short a time. They are so terrified of doing without food for 18 hours that these patients, fortunately only a few, have either refused or quit my program, rather than carry out this test. For the vast majority who do go through with the semi-fast overnight, there is no question as to the benefit. A new confidence can be seen building in their minds. They find that delaying or skipping a meal or snack is not the ultimate disaster. They do not die and they suffer no ill effects.

This prepares them for any situation in which they are unable to eat properly or must delay getting the right foods or have a choice between eating problem foods and waiting a short interval for a better selection of things to eat and drink. This short exercise is one of the most potent builders of strength in dieting that I know of.

Another good way to build proficiency and confidence is to have the dieter name his or her favorite food or treat. It should be something almost irresistible to that person. Have the second or third most problematic item listed as well. Get the dieter to buy each item and place a triple portion of each on a plate, in a glass, or in a bowl. The next step is to sit down in front of one or more of these at a time, pick up a spoon or fork and place one tiny sample into the mouth. Do not swallow it! Hold the sample in the mouth for a full minute by carefully looking at a watch and measuring the time. The next paragraph lists the instructions following a minute's wait.

Feel the texture, if any, of the food. Let your tongue taste all of the different flavors present. See if you can separate out these flavors. After a minute, swallow the portion you placed in your mouth. Put your fork or spoon down and get up from the table. Let the food sit there for three hours and then place it in the garbage or disposal unit of your sink. Write down your feelings about what you have done with these three favorite foods and bring them in on your next visit to this office.

Another useful exercise in controlling hunger is to widen the range of foods that a dieter will eat. Vegetables, salads, soups, and most fruits are almost foreign substances to many problem eaters. I usually suggest one new food every third day. A new vegetable or fruit is eaten in at least two different ways over that time. The food is placed in the mouth, chewed slowly, the flavors are savored and analyzed by the dieter, and a decision is made as to whether the food is really "bad" or not. On the initial interview and history we ask about foods that are avoided and a list is made. The foods that are thought to be tasteless, dull, or foreign to the patient are listed, and a program of reintroducing these into a reducing or maintenance diet is discussed, provided the food is wholesome and desirable.

A much greater variety of foods is encouraged through this experimentation into new or previously rejected items. Boredom is a constant threat to dietary compliance, so these new and sometimes surprisingly good-tasting dishes can help fill out what might have become a monotonous routine of only a relatively few different foods.

In summary, true hunger is rare. We all are storehouses of ten-thousands of calories of usable energy. The real discomfort we feel when we try to lose weight is a learned one. Getting in touch with our true feelings and learning what the body, mind, and spirit are really saying is the initial goal for all who want a healthy and slim body. Part of the next chapter also deals with hunger and appetite.

The keys to permanent weight loss and health are self-knowledge, self-love, self-forgiveness, and self-respect. Attain these and the slim body follows as a natural and comfortably attained result.

CHAPTER TWELVE

THINGS THAT NEED TO BE SAID

This chapter is made up of a group of suggestions that I have used in my practice for the past several decades. They are hints about different things, and I hope they will be of some use to you in handling a certain problem or in understanding the process of weight and fat loss. In many cases I may have mentioned something about some of these techniques in another part of the book. I believe in repetition to reinforce what might have been previously covered. It is a valuable teaching tool.

HUNGER AND APPETITE

Most dieters are unable to distinguish between appetite and true hunger. Most of their problem eating is a result of habits, environmental influences, and emotional stress. Provided a person has eaten an adequate amount of food to satisfy true hunger, and provided there are no real or imagined hypoglycemic episodes from unwise eating a few hours before, there should be no real hunger experienced until four or five hours after a meal.

I have asked many patients who complained of hunger how each one feels when he or she is hungry. If weakness is the symptom and nothing else, it could be caused by hypoglycemia or pseudohypoglycemia (low or imagined low blood sugar). There are those who feel that hypoglycemia is not a real entity in medicine, but whatever you might call it, if a person becomes jittery, weak, irritable, or ravenously hungry a few hours after a trigger substance is consumed, it makes little difference what it is called. Usually removing the sugar, alcohol, or excess caffeine from that person's diet will result in disappearance of the symptoms.

Another common sensation interpreted as hunger is a feeling of emptiness, gnawing, rumbling, or actual pain in the "stomach" area. When one considers that the stomach is only supposed to be "full" three or four times a day at most, the thought that it should never be kept empty seems ridiculous. It is estimated that the stomach is empty of food about 70 to 80 per cent of the time, with little or no harmful effects.

If a dieter is used to immediately putting food into her stomach whenever there is rumbling or burning, the entire process of slimming is compromised. Even if relatively strong hunger suppressants are used, the feedback loop of "stomach filling" cannot be bypassed, and failure on the program results. Only with education can a patient be convinced to take in antacids or low-calorie soups to ease the discomfort of what is probably stress-produced excess acidity and stomach spasms.

Many overweight patients have what are called hiatal hernias, or weaknesses in the area of the diaphragm where the esophagus passes through on the way to the upper stomach. Backsurges of stomach acid can cause distress and a tendency to eat to relieve the pain. Fortunately, the prime treatment for this type of hernia is weight loss, combined with medications to control acid production or neutralize excess acid. If weight is lost, the symptoms get better. The problem lies in the uneducated patient who treats her problem with the very thing that will make it worse, fat-producing excess calories. The key remedy is education of patients to avoid the wrong response to what a stomach is "telling" them.

I have had patients tell me that vitamins made them hungry. This is usually not the case, but you will possibly have an argument on your hands unless you convince the patient that he or she is wrong. Vitamins and minerals can be quite irritating to the stomach. This irritation can be as bad sometimes as excess acid. The patient feels discomfort and automatically turns to food as the cure-all for the queasy or nauseated feeling. Some of the patients tell me it is to "settle the stomach," but I usually remind them that the stomach is too "settled" already and is overlapping his or her belt in some cases. The solution is not to argue with the patient but to convince him or her to take the vitamins, etc., with food. Right in the middle of the largest meal of the day is better. If one brand doesn't agree, in spite of taking it with food, try another, but try and make sure that you don't go without the needed support that these supplements give you.

Another trigger to problem eating is habit. This can be overcome by a process of reconditioning the patient to respond in a more appropriate manner when certain stimuli are encountered. Feeding a habit makes it thrive while starving it will eventually kill it. The way to totally destroy a bad habit is to replace it with a good habit. Much has been written in the psychological literature about behavior modification. It has been accused of being a failure for long-term treatment, and perhaps this could be partly true if that is all that is used.

The key seems to be a *comprehensive* program that also includes exercise and good dietary practices to overcome the Set Point. Knowledge of what actually goes on in the body is one of the most powerful forces to use against your obesity. In other parts of this book you will see these processes described, so take advantage of this learning opportunity and go past the search for the quick fix for overweight in order to concentrate on permanent slimness.

The next time you feel that you are hungry, take a good mental look inside your body and analyze your feelings objectively. Is it food or antacid that you need? How long has it been since you had a good meal? Have you had any sweets, alcohol, or excess caffeine in the past two to five hours? Are you nervous, annoyed, tired, sad, or excessively happy or excited? Does this feeling usually make you eat? If you resorted to delaying tactics, would this feeling of wanting, rather than needing, food go away? It doesn't take long before you can become knowledgeable about your own internal and external feelings, and this knowledge can make you able to say NO to your body when it tries to trick you into eating unwisely.

GUILT VERSUS REALISM IN WEIGHT REDUCTION

You are learning a skill when you attempt to change your way of dealing with food and problem eating habits. Like the learning of any other skill, there are often mistakes associated with the process. Too many patients are destroyed by their errors and are triggered to go on an eating binge when they have only experienced a single problem. If you were learning math, you wouldn't let a few troubles make you quit the course? Of course not! So why let an episode of problem eating ruin your diet program?

This is a form of Self-Defeating Behavior (SDB), and is quite common in the dieting population. SDB occurs when a patient doesn't have the proper insight into what makes him or her behave in a certain way. Going off a diet program, even a little bit, sets off an orgy of guilt, self-accusation, and self-punishment. The punishment is usually in the form of quitting slimming efforts altogether, or going on a short binge. The self-abuse with food is followed by even more guilt, feelings of helplessness, and more eating. The only thing that can break the cycle is the attainment of awareness of the process by the patient.

Rule number one in conquering SDB is to be realistic about what you are trying to do. Your primary goal isn't to lose weight, it is to change your eating habits. An extra pound of water weight on the scale can throw many of you off your programs for no valid reason at all. You are letting a few pints of temporary water gain ruin all your efforts. I have seen patients who were losing fat rapidly, but who also temporarily accumulated extra water weight, go into hysterics, and cry over what a scale told them, instead of what their minds and their loose clothing should have been telling them.

If you find yourself deviating from your slimming program, don't just say, "To Hell with it, I might as well just eat all I want today!" Go right back on the program *then*; don't binge.

Another form of SDB is to ignore the vast amount of data that supports the use of a diary in your program. A lot of dieters have excuses for not bringing in a diary for monitoring. "I don't have *time* to bother with that diary." "I don't think you trust me." "I wouldn't *dare* bring you in a diary with what I eat every day. I would be ashamed to."

None of these rather weak excuses really justifies not sharing your pattern of eating with your therapist. In fact, we know that if everything else is equal, patients who bring in a diary weekly are twice as likely to be successful as those who don't. That's a powerful argument in favor of the diary. In spite of this, many patients either refuse to bring it, or conveniently "forget" it week after week.

In my practice, my rule of letting realism be my goal in the office makes me gently try to get these "lost sheep" to bring in their diaries, at the risk of making them angry. Why would I continue to insist on having another pair of eyes and ears through reading the diary, particularly when I know it generates anger in some people? The reason is obvious. I feel it would help you to do better, especially if your weight or size is stuck and there is no movement downward.

These are only a few of the SDB patterns that I observe in my patients. Don't look at your therapist as a parent figure who will punish and shame you if a mistake is made. Look at the relationship as a partnership, with each party contributing his or her efforts toward your ultimate success.

MOTIVATIONAL ROADBLOCKS

Most people who are overweight are very unhappy about their obesity. So why do they have so much trouble starting a diet program, or sticking to it? I believe that would-be dieters succumb to a variety of motivational roadblocks. Let's consider several of these and suggest how you can steer your way around them.

Let's start with the almost universal feeling among dieters that their being on a diet is somehow (cost-wise, time-wise, etc.) unfair to their families. However, the truth is that what's really unfair to their loved ones is remaining overweight. This is because of the risk involved of developing any number of serious, life-threatening diseases. If you have ever felt guilty, for example, about spending money to lose weight, ask yourself the following question: "What do my children need more, new designer jeans, or a healthy me who will be alive and well to love and nurture them?" Really at issue is not whether you can afford to lose weight, but whether you can afford not to.

Another reason many people have difficulty starting a diet, or sticking to it, relates to their history of previous diet failures. Individuals who have tried unsuccessfully to diet many times in the past may be convinced that to try again would only mean having to face failure one more time. They may also feel that they will receive ridicule from their families and friends if they even suggest that they are going on a diet "one more time." These individuals have convinced themselves (or have been convinced by others) that they will always be fat because they have no willpower or self-control. However, these same people often display considerable willpower and great self-control in other areas of their lives.

For example, in their role as parent, they are able to get up in the middle of the night to care for a sick child, even when they themselves are feeling ill. Doesn't such behavior require willpower and self-control?

These individuals should now recognize that their failures to diet successfully in the past were not matters of their lacking willpower or self-control. The real "culprit" was a lack of knowledge about how to avoid or lessen the impact of such dieting pitfalls as weight loss plateaus, binges, and the feelings of deprivation, fatigue, and boredom. In the absence of such knowledge, dieting can be a frustrating and highly stressful experience. This is why dieters should seek some sort of motivational help rather than continually try to diet on their own.

It isn't only people who have unsuccessfully dieted in the past who encounter motivational roadblocks. Individuals who have histories of successful dieting but unsuccessful maintenance are also frequently reluctant to start a new diet program. They tend to feel that even if they once again take the weight off, it will return again, sometimes with interest. Their concern is *justified*! However, they need to understand that the main reason dieters put weight back on is that dieting alone does *nothing* to change the habits and patterns which were responsible for the excess fat in the first place.

Thus, if you have repeatedly lost and regained excess poundage, there is cause for hope, as well as concern. You can learn how to change your habit patterns and make your next diet a *lasting* success.

If you can perceive how you might now be able to steer around the motivational roadblock I've described, why not make a new start? Are you thinking to yourself: "I will, but right now I'm too busy?" If you are thinking that, you've just run into another roadblock! There will always be stressful and busy times in life, and these are probably the very times when you will most likely overeat and gain weight. Now is the time to learn techniques for coping with stress in non-food ways. Such techniques are mentioned in another part of this booklet. Why not start now?

DEALING WITH PESTS AND FEEDER-SABOTEURS

Many patients report that relatives and so-called "friends" will attempt to get them to eat by trying to talk them into it. Below are a couple of simulated conversations with these pests in certain situations. It would pay you to do a little CR when alone, so that when these occur, you are primed and ready to defend yourself.

1) The "Who, me?" approach. When told that you should stop losing weight and get off "that diet" before it kills you (this is when you are still 50 pounds overweight), and that you should eat more, say the following or something similar with the most innocent tone you can manage without laughing in his or her face:

Who, me? Do you really think I'm thinner? Honestly, I haven't really thought about it. Why are you concerned? I'm not on a diet. (It's an eating program, so you're telling the truth.)

Gee! I guess I am a little smaller, but I wouldn't let it worry you. By the way, what is the purpose in your bringing up something like this to me. I always consider what I weigh and what I eat as a highly personal thing, like my sex life. Incidentally, how *is* yours?

It's interesting that you should bring up my weight. I had been a little worried about *you*! You're looking a little pale and sickly lately. Is everything alright with you? Have you seen your doctor lately for an AIDS or a cancer checkup? (This last comes under the rule that the best defense is a good offense.)

Use all or part of the above, or something similar.

2) The Broken Record, or Parrot Technique. When offered food that you don't want, continue to repeat the same phrase over and over again while still agreeing with the pest. This is a powerful rejection technique that I learned from one of my mentors in Bariatrics, the late Peter G. Lindner, M.D.

Pest: Have some cake.

You: Thank you, but I just don't care for it.

Pest: But you always did like cake.

You: You're right, but now I just don't care for it.

Pest: It's not that many calories and it really won't mess you up on your diet.

You: I suppose that you're correct, but I just don't care for it.

Pest: I wish you'd get off that diet.

You: You could be right, if I were on a diet, but I just don't care for it.

Pest: You're not being very friendly by not eating my cake after I made it *just for you*!

You: I suppose you might assume that, but I really don't care for any.

At this point the pest leaves to find another victim. Remember, don't admit you're on a diet and don't use the fact that you're dieting as justification. You don't *need* to justify your actions to anyone. If you use the diet as a reason not to eat the (whatever), the pest will want to know all about it and will argue that in her professional (unofficial doctor) opinion, the cake is no problem. It isn't a problem for *her*, but it *will* be for you if you give in. I have used cake as an example, but it could be any food or group of foods that might tempt you.

For those of you who are not yet ready to confront a pest directly, there is always another approach. State that whatever food you are being offered by the pest doesn't agree with you. You aren't saying you are allergic to it, or that it makes you sick. You are just saying that it doesn't agree with you. In a way, this is correct. If you ate or drank the problem food or beverage, you would be off your program and probably gaining weight in the bargain. In this sense it doesn't agree with you.

WHAT ARE YOU REALLY LOSING WHEN YOU DIET?

This section will *really* sound like repetition of what was said earlier. Forgive this, but what is written here, if understood, can markedly influence whether or not you are ultimately a success at attaining normal weight.

What is it that you hope you lose when you go on a diet? The answer is weight, of course, but the weight of what? Each person's overall weight is composed of two components. One of these consists of the individual's muscles, bones, and vital organ tissues. It, along with the body water, is called the lean body mass (LBM). The other component is fat. Although most people talk about wanting to lose weight, are you *really* interested in losing muscles and other vital tissues, or are you trying to lose fat?

Unless you have a weight clause in your work contract, like some airline employees have, you really shouldn't be concerned with your weight at all. Rather, you should be concerned about whether or not you have excess fat deposited on your body. After all, it is excess fat that jeopardizes your health and detracts from your appearance. If you think about it, have you heard anybody complain lately that their muscles were too heavy?

It is known that if we diet without exercising, we lose too high a proportion of LBM, along with the fat. Since it isn't healthy to lose vital tissue over a period of time, this loss of mostly muscle protein must be minimized. If we aren't careful this muscle loss can be substantial. Charles Kuntzelman, author of the book *Diet Free*, contends that for every pound of fat we lose, we *could* lose as much as two pounds of LBM. The fat loss is desirable, but the muscle loss is not. That's because the more muscle tissue we have, the more calories we require to maintain the same weight.

While dieting without exercise can result in the loss of a substantial amount of muscle as well as fat, I'm happy to report that if you exercise properly while dieting, about 90 per cent or more of the weight you lose will be fat. If you're wondering how it's possible to tell whether the weight the person is losing is fat or muscle LBM, the answer lies in weighing the individual under water, using at least two separate measurements.

The person undergoing underwater weighing submerges himself or herself in a tank of water while breathing through snorkeling equipment. The measurements taken of water displacement and body density while the person is submerged permit a relatively precise assessment of the individual's percentage of body fat. What percentage is desirable? Relying, in part, on studies of the exact body composition of various deceased subjects, exercise physiologists tend to recommend about 20 to 27 per cent body fat for women, and 13 to 20 per cent for men.

With these percentages in mind, an individual can learn from being weighed underwater what his or her "ideal weight" is.

Suppose, for instance, that a 150-pound woman learned from being weighed under water that she has 100 pounds of lean body mass and 50 pounds of fat, or a body composed of 33 per cent fat. If she wants to get down to 20 per cent fat, her ideal weight, given her 100 pounds of LBM, would be 125 pounds. This supposes 25 pounds of fat out of 125, or 20 per cent.

If you decide you are interested in having your percentage of body fat determined by underwater weighing, contact your local medical school or university with a sportsmedicine department for further details. Even if you're not interested in that, do think more in terms of body composition than you do about body weight. Remember, if you don't exercise, your loss of body weight may be actually indicative of a detrimental change in body composition.

Unfortunately, the only form of exercise practiced by some dieters is hopping on and off the scale. Do you live in fear of the scale? How many days have been ruined for you because the scale showed that you gained an ounce or two? If you have understood what I have been discussing up to this point, you should be able to free yourself from enslavement by the scale. Begin by *repeatedly* reminding yourself that your concern is with losing fat, rather than weight. Then develop the habit of gauging your dieting progress in terms of changes that reflect loss of FAT, such as a shrinkage in your body measurements and a need for smaller sizes of clothing.

It is also important that you realize that a slower than expected loss, or actual gain of body weight, may indicate a beneficial change in body composition. What I am referring to is the fact that when they diet and exercise, some patients actually GAIN lean body mass. If you are losing inches like crazy, but the scale isn't budging, don't worry about it. It means a loss of fat and a gain of valuable LBM. Your friends will all assume that you have lost "weight" because of your slimmer look. If they ask you how much you've lost, simply say: "I've gone from a size — — to a size — —.

In order to lose fat and not LBM, you MUST incorporate an exercise habit into your daily routine. To find out about the proper aerobic exercises and the proper way to do them daily (pulse monitoring), read the excellent paperback book *Fit or Fat*, by Covert Baily.

You will notice no extensive chapter on exercise in this book. There is a reason for this. I prefer for exercise to be gentle and progressively more difficult. Walking is the best of all exercises for dieters. There is less likelihood of injury to you and it takes very little equipment.

Work up to walking three or more miles a day at a pace of from 15 to 20 minutes per mile. Most of you should not try jogging or running. There is just too much difficulty and potential for injury in anything other than a walk.

Below are my calculations as to what physical activity burns for a 30-minute exercise session. Values are for a 70 kg (154 pound) person. No distinction is made for the sex of the exerciser. Persons weighing more will probably burn more, but this is the minimum caloric cost of the exercises per 30 minutes:

Badminton	**200**
Cycling, a mile in 11 minutes	**130**
Cycling, a mile in 6.4 minutes	**210**
Dancing, easy and moderate tempo	**110**
Dancing, aerobic type	**350**
Gymnastics	**140**
Horseback riding at trot	**230**
Judo or Karate, katas and workout	**400**
Minitrampoline or rebounder, 100 to 120 steps per minute, low jogging	**130**
Minitramp — higher step	**200**
Pingpong, singles	**140**
Rowing machine, moderate pace	**150**
Running, 11 minute mile	**300**
Running, 9 minute mile	**410**
Running, 6 minute mile	**525**
Skiing, downhill	**250**
Skiing, cross country	**300**
Fitness Master	**250 to 300**

Squash	440
Stair climbing, up, 60 steps/minute	430
Stair climbing, down, same rate	100
Swimming laps, moderate pace	270
Swimming laps, racing speed	330
Tennis, singles	225
Walking, 20 minute mile	130
Walking, 15 minute mile	200

You will notice that if you were to walk for thirty minutes every day at a pace of four miles an hour, you could expend enough extra calories every 18 days to lose an extra pound. This would add up to about 20 pounds of fat lost a year if everything else was kept constant. See your therapist and work out an exercise program prior to going on it. Be sure your medical condition is such that walking or some other exercise is not a problem for you.

HOW TO FAIL AT THE WEIGHT LOSS GAME!

The last item in this booklet is a negative way of telling you how to succeed, as you shall see. A lot of my patients want to know how to fail at losing weight. Believe me, it's easy! Just do all the things I list in this section, or even part of them, and you should have no problem keeping your fat deposits. Also, in the event you want to SUCCEED, just do the OPPOSITE of what I say below.

1) Listen to all your friends when they tell you that you don't need to lose any more weight. After all, they are experts and many of them have medical degrees, don't they? They have no reasons, such as jealousy or envy, that would make them say something like this. Even if you are five feet tall and weigh 180 pounds, it pays to listen to fools who would sabotage your efforts to improve your health and well-being.
2) Rely strictly on your "appetite suppressants" to do all the work for you. Ignore the massive amount of medical research that has shown that these medications by themselves are only

marginally useful as a temporary measure in controlling hunger and adjusting the Set Point and have no long-term effect. Be sure you don't build up a bunch of good habits to replace the bad ones that helped make you overweight in the first place.

3) When you go to a party or social function, be sure to starve yourself before going so that you are ravenous enough and vulnerable enough to "pig out" after you get there. In order to fail properly and completely, be sure not to eat enough to keep you out of trouble BEFORE you leave home or work to go there.

4) If you have them, be sure to take your diuretics (water pills) more often than the directions say. Use them to take off "weight" rather than excess edema fluid. Don't worry about the potentially dangerous side-effects that can occur if they are taken too often. Also, be sure to load up on forbidden foods that are high in sodium (salt), so that you can bloat up again tomorrow. Don't tell your therapist about your medicines prescribed by other doctors, including diuretics and heart drugs, that you are taking. It would only confuse the poor man and keep him from giving you some of the ones he uses.

5) If you make a mistake, be sure to heap a lot of guilt on yourself. A little guilt will go a long way. Once you have made that one mistake, tell yourself that since you have already blown it, you may as well stay off the diet for the rest of the month. Be sure to deny any problems on your next visit to the therapist. Don't share the problems that have come up with him or her and the clinic staff.

6) Become a "COUCH POTATO" and *never* exercise because it could become habit-forming. Do as little moving around as possible and never take the stairs or park more than a few feet away from a store. Be sure to park in the handicapped spaces and run into the store wearing your tennis outfit or jogging suit.

7) Let your problems, anxieties, anger, sadness, or depression make you eat. It is better to crush bad feelings underneath a load of food than to deal with them in an adult manner. Get inside your shell or closet and EAT!

8) Be sure *not* to take your vitamins and minerals if they are prescribed for you. They might make you hungry! Ignore the evidence that vitamins don't increase appetite if they are formulated correctly. Don't take a chance. All that those vitamins and minerals do is to stimulate the chemical machinery that helps your fat burning system work better.

9) Don't read the information in this book, or anything that your therapist gives you. Instead, look in the *Enquirer* for the latest miracle diet and eat what it says to, plus whatever else you want.

There are other "helpful hints" that I could list, but it should be obvious to all of you that these keys to failure are not things you should really be doing. They were listed in this negative way to get your attention.

I told you at the beginning of this chapter that it would be a miscellaneous group of items and I hope you were able to get something out of them. They are meant to stimulate your thought processes and get you to change certain behaviors and ways of dealing with your environment. There are other items in other parts of this booklet that I have found useful for over 20 years with my own patients.

The most efficient way to utilize these bits and pieces of information is to read over each of them at least once a month. Each time you read them you will see something new, or it will strike you in a slightly different way. By this repetition you will grow in strength of will and habit, eventually reaching your goal of permanent slimness.

CHAPTER THIRTEEN

CONVENIENCE FOODS AND THEIR USE IN A MAINTENANCE DIET

It is quite possible to enjoy the easily prepared frozen or pre-packaged foods and still stay on a maintenance diet. It is better not to use this kind of food until you are off a weight reduction program because of the relatively high caloric content of some of the foods. In addition to the usual foods that are prepared relatively quickly, I want to cover a few of the regular foods and their starch content. It makes little sense to add something to your daily intake thinking it is a starch and later find out it was almost all sugar. For this reason we have a relatively large amount of foodstuffs to classify in this chapter for your convenience.

HOW TO USE THE EXCHANGE TABLES FOR CONVENIENCE FOODS

These tables of food values for certain convenience foods are for the use of a person who is dieting to keep at a certain weight. Diabetics on insulin should know that these values are usually only an approximation. The values are good enough for everyone else in order to show what the food content is. If in doubt, consult your local bariatric physician, diabetes specialist, or consulting nutritionist.

The values are given in terms of the equivalent amount of bread, lean meat, fat, milk, vegetable, or fruit exchanges in a portion specified by the manufacturer or designated here. An exchange of a particular food group may also be called a portion. The two words are interchangeable. For example, a bread exchange or portion may be a slice of bread, or the equivalent amount of starchy food found in a potato, in a helping of rice, or in a helping of beans. Each of these is the same as far as food value is concerned and they may be exchanged for each other and not upset a diet. This is where the word "exchange" comes from. A separate section is included on cereals. It is useful to know how much of the cereal is starch and related carbohydrates, and how much is sugar.

Sources for these values were partly from the companies, partly from the package labeling, and partly from my own calculations. Alcoholic beverages are included in this section for your information, even though these are empty calories, for the sake of completeness.

Be aware of the following measurements used commonly:

> One tablespoon equals three teaspoons.
> Two tablespoons equals one ounce.
> Four ounces equals one-half cup.
> Eight ounces equals one cup.

Take the particular caloric intake diet that you are on and study how much of each food group is permitted each day. Fit the convenience foods into your daily intake carefully. It seems hard now, but it becomes easier every day you do it.

At the end of the chapter is a special group of foods listed according to the manufacturer. They are listed according to the number of calories in the food, but also may have either the diabetic exchange (portion) information or the amount of protein, carbohydrate, and fat present. There are two ways you can calculate the foods listed here. These two methods are listed along with the amounts to be deducted from the daily ration of foods and/or calories.

The manufacturers listed in the special end-of-chapter list are Benihana, Candle Lite, Classic Lite, Dining Lite, Lean Cuisine, Light & Elegant, and Weight Watchers. All of the entrees listed here contain 300 calories or less, and are for the use of slimmers who wish to have the convenience of a quickly-prepared frozen meal without the bother of fixing it from scratch. All food values are approximate and are intended for the use of persons trying to limit their calories, either to lose weight or to maintain it once the desired weight is reached. The values given in these tables being approximate ones, they are not meant for diabetics or others who must have exact proportions.

ALCOHOLIC BEVERAGES

The alcoholic beverages listed here are not all the ones that exist. In cases of mixed drinks that I haven't listed here, take the basic ingredients and calculate the exchanges from that data. Alcohol is "burned" by the body similarly to fats, so we consider it in that category. This means for each 45 calories of alcohol we must give up one fat portion (exchange) for that day. The other components of mixed drinks are usually sugar, so we omit one fruit portion for each 40 calories, or 10 grams, of carbohydrate. The drinks listed below are listed in terms of their fat and fruit equivalents.

TYPE OF DRINK AND/OR BRAND	MEASURE USED FOR BEVERAGE	EXCHANGE INFORMATION
Ale, Mild	8 ounces	1½ fat, 1 fruit
Beer	8 ounces	1½ fat, 1 fruit
WINES		
Champagne, Brut	3 ounces	1⅔ fat
Champagne, Extra Dry	3 ounces	1⅔ fat, ½ fruit

Dubonnet	3 ounces	$1\frac{1}{2}$ fat, 1 fruit
Dry Marsala	3 ounces	2 fats, 2 fruits
Sweet Marsala	3 ounces	2 fats, $2\frac{1}{2}$ fruits
Muscatel	4 ounces	$2\frac{1}{3}$ fats, $1\frac{1}{2}$ fruits
Port	4 ounces	$2\frac{1}{3}$ fats, $1\frac{1}{2}$ fruits
Dry Red Wine	3 ounces	$1\frac{2}{3}$ fats
Sake	3 ounces	1 fat, 1 fruit
Domestic Sherry	$3\frac{1}{2}$ ounces	$1\frac{1}{2}$ fats, $\frac{1}{2}$ fruit
Dry Vermouth	$3\frac{1}{2}$ ounces	$2\frac{1}{3}$ fats
Sweet Vermouth	$3\frac{1}{2}$ ounces	$2\frac{2}{3}$ fats, 1 fruit
Dry White Wine	3 ounces	$1\frac{1}{2}$ fats

LIQUEURS AND CORDIALS

Amaretto	1 ounce	$1\frac{1}{3}$ fats, $1\frac{1}{2}$ fruits
Creme de Cacao	1 ounce	$1\frac{1}{2}$ fats, 1 fruit
Creme de Menthe	1 ounce	$1\frac{1}{2}$ fats, 1 fruit
Curacao	1 ounce	$1\frac{1}{2}$ fats, 1 fruit
Drambuie	1 ounce	$1\frac{1}{2}$ fats, 1 fruit
Tia Maria	1 ounce	$1\frac{1}{2}$ fats, 1 fruit

SPIRITS

Bourbon, brandy, cognac, Canadian whiskey, gin, rye, rum, Scotch, tequila, and vodka are essentially free of carbohydrates. Caloric or fat portion count depends on the proof. Values are rounded off.

80 proof	1 ounce	$1\frac{1}{2}$ fats
84 proof	1 ounce	$1\frac{1}{2}$ fats
90 proof	1 ounce	$1\frac{2}{3}$ fats
94 proof	1 ounce	2 fats
97 proof	1 ounce	2 fats
100 proof	1 ounce	$2\frac{1}{4}$ fats

There are a lot more alcoholic beverages that are not covered here, but these are some of the more popular ones. It is well to remember that alcohol seems to impede the progress of a dieter for many reasons. Alcohol seems to help the fat making "machinery" in our bodies and slow down the fat burning mechanisms. In a lot of dieters it also causes increased appetite, not your ideal situation. The best course of action is to drink as little alcohol as possible while dieting and drink in moderation after the ideal goal is reached. Remember, if you drink alcohol, calculate the portions you have consumed and keep track of them.

CANNED AND PACKAGED FOODS

BRAND NAME	MEASURE USED FOR FOOD	EXCHANGE INFORMATION
Alba 77, Fit 'N Frosty Drink, any flavor	1 envelope	1 low-fat milk
Aunt Penny's Cheese Sauce	2 Tablespoons	$^1/_2$ meat and $^1/_2$ cooked vegetable
Aunt Penny's Hollandaise Sauce	2 Tablespoons	Same
Aunt Penny's White Sauce	2 Tablespoons	Same
BANQUET BRAND		
Beef Stew	8 ounces	2 breads and 1 meat
Chicken and Dumplings	8 ounces	2 breads and 3 meats
Creamed Chipped Beef	5 ounces	1 meat and 2 cooked vegetables
Salisbury Steak with Gravy	5 ounces	2 meats, 1 cooked vegetable, 1 fat
Spaghetti with Meat Sauce	8 ounces	2 meats, 3 fruits, 1 fat
BETTY CROCKER		
Macaroni and Cheddar	$^1/_2$ cup	1 bread and 1 fat
Noodles Almondine	$^1/_2$ cup	1 bread, 1 milk, $^1/_2$ fat
Noodles Italiano	$^1/_2$ cup	1 bread, $^1/_2$ milk
Noodles Romanoff	$^1/_2$ cup	1 bread, 1 milk, $^1/_2$ fat
Chili-Tomato Hamburger Helper Mix	$^1/_5$ package	2 breads, $^1/_2$ fat
Hamburger Helper Mix	$^1/_5$ package	$1^1/_2$ breads, trace fat
Lasagna Hamburger Helper Mix	$^1/_5$ package	2 breads
Spaghetti Hamburger Helper Mix	$^1/_5$ package	2 breads
Cheeseburger Macaroni Hamburger Helper Mix	$^1/_5$ package	2 breads, 1 fat
Rice Milanese	$^1/_2$ cup	2 breads, $1^1/_2$ fats
Rice Provence	$^1/_2$ cup	2 breads, $^1/_2$ fat
Creamy Noodles 'n Tuna or Hamburger Helper Mix	$^1/_5$ package	2 breads, 2 fats
Creamy Rice 'n Tuna or Hamburger Helper Mix	$^1/_5$ package	2 breads, 1 fat
Dry Hash Brown Potato Mix	$^1/_4$ package	3 breads
Dry Scalloped Potato Mix	$^1/_4$ package	3 breads
Instant Mashed Potato Buds	$^1/_2$ cup	$1^1/_2$ breads

BIRDS EYE BRAND

Awake Imitation Orange Juice	¹/₂ cup	1¹/₂ fruits
Bavarian-style Beans with Spaetzle	¹/₂ cup	2 vegetables
Broccoli Spears in butter sauce	¹/₂ cup	¹/₂ vegetable and 1 fat
Broccoli with cheese sauce	¹/₂ cup	2 vegetables and 2 fats
Broccoli, Carrots and Pasta Twists	¹/₂ cup	¹/₂ bread, 1 vegetable, 1 fat
Carrots with brown sugar glaze	¹/₂ cup	1 fruit, 1 vegetable, ¹/₂ fat
Chinese-style Vegetables	¹/₂ cup	1 vegetable
Cook Whip Nondairy Topping	2 Tablespoons	¹/₄ milk
Corn in butter sauce	¹/₂ cup	1 bread and 1 fat
Corn, Green Beans & Pasta Curls	¹/₂ cup	1 bread, 1 vegetable, 1 fat
Corn, Peas, and Tomatoes	¹/₂ cup	2 vegetables
French-style Green Beans with Almonds	¹/₂ cup	1 vegetable, ¹/₂ fat
French-style Green Beans with Mushrooms	¹/₂ cup	1 vegetable
French-style Rice	¹/₂ cup	1¹/₂ bread, 1 vegetable
Green Beans in cream sauce	¹/₂ cup	¹/₂ bread, 1 vegetable, 1¹/₂ fats
Green Peas and Onions	¹/₂ cup	2 vegetables
Green Peas in butter sauce	¹/₂ cup	1¹/₂ vegetables, 1 fat
Green Peas and Celery	¹/₂ cup	1¹/₂ vegetables
Green Peas and Mushrooms	¹/₂ cup	1¹/₂ vegetables
Italian-style Vegetables	¹/₂ cup	2 vegetables
Italian-style Rice	¹/₂ cup	1 vegetable, 1¹/₂ breads
Japanese-style Vegetables	¹/₂ cup	2 vegetables
Mixed Vegetables with onion sauce	¹/₂ cup	1 vegetable, ¹/₂ bread, 1 fat
New England-style Vegetables	¹/₂ cup	2 vegetables
Oriental-style Rice	¹/₂ cup	1 vegetable, 1¹/₂ breads
Peas, Shells, and Corn	¹/₂ cup	1 vegetable, 1 bread, 1 fat
Peas, Shells, and Mushrooms	¹/₂ cup	1 vegetable, 1 bread, 1 fat
Pennsylvania Dutch-style Vegetables	¹/₂ cup	1¹/₂ vegetables
Rice and Peas with Mushrooms	¹/₂ cup	1 vegetable, 1 bread
San Francisco-style Vegetables	¹/₂ cup	2 vegetables
Spanish-style Rice	¹/₂ cup	1 vegetable, 1¹/₂ breads
Creamed Spinach	¹/₂ cup	1 vegetable, 1 fat

Wisconsin Country-style Vegetables	¹/₂ **cup**	1¹/₂ **vegetables**
Crinkle or Plain French Fried Potatoes	3 **oz. (1 serving)**	1¹/₂ **breads, 1 fat**
Potato Pattie	3 **oz. (1 serving)**	1 **bread, 2 fats**
Potato Puffs	¹/₃ **package**	1 **bread, 2 fats**
Hash Browns	¹/₂ **cup**	1 **bread**
Onion Rings	2 **oz. (¹/₂ sm.pkg.) or 2 oz. (¹/₃ lg. pkg.)**	1 **bread, 2 fats**

BOUNTY (CAMPBELL'S)

Beef Stew	1 **cup**	1 **bread, 2 meats**
Chicken Stew	1 **cup**	1 **bread, 1¹/₂ meats**
Chili Con Carne with Beans	1 **cup**	1 **bread, 1 meat**

CAMPBELL'S CONDENSED SOUPS
(All servings ¹/₂ can, given in number of prepared ounces)

Asparagus, Cream of	10 **ounces**	1 **bread, 1 fat**
Bean with Bacon	11 **ounces**	2 **breads, ¹/₂ meat, 1 fat**
Beef	11 **ounces**	1 **bread, 1 meat**
Beef Broth (bouillon)	10 **ounces**	**Free Food**
Beef Broth and Barley	11 **ounces**	1 **bread, ¹/₂ fat**
Beef Broth and Noodles	10 **ounces**	1 **bread, ¹/₂ fat**
Beef Noodle	10 **ounces**	1 **bread, ¹/₂ fat**
Beef Teriyaki	10 **ounces**	1 **bread, ¹/₂ meat**
Beefy Mushroom	10 **ounces**	¹/₂ **bread, 1 meat**
Black Bean	11 **ounces**	1¹/₂ **bread, ¹/₂ meat**
Celery, Cream of	10 **ounces**	¹/₂ **bread, 2 fats**
Cheddar Cheese	11 **ounces**	1 **milk, 2 fats**
Chicken Alphabet	10 **ounces**	1 **bread, ¹/₂ fat**
Chicken Broth	10 **ounces**	1 **meat**
Chicken Broth and Noodles	10 **ounces**	¹/₂ **bread, 1 fat**
Chicken Broth and Rice	10 **ounces**	1 **bread**
Chicken Broth and Vegetables	10 **ounces**	¹/₂ **bread**
Chicken, Cream of	10 **ounces**	¹/₂ **bread, 2 fats**
Chicken 'n Dumplings	10 **ounces**	¹/₂ **bread, ¹/₂ meat, 1 fat**
Chicken Gumbo	10 **ounces**	1 **bread**
Chicken Noodle	10 **ounces**	1 **bread, ¹/₂ fat**
Chicken NoodleO's	10 **ounces**	1 **bread, ¹/₂ fat**
Chicken with Rice	10 **ounces**	¹/₂ **bread, 1 fat**
Chicken and Stars	10 **ounces**	¹/₂ **bread, 1 fat**
Chicken Vegetable	10 **ounces**	1 **bread, ¹/₂ fat**
Chili Beef	11 **ounces**	1¹/₂ **breads, 1 meat, ¹/₂ fat**
Clam Chowder (Manhattan)	10 **ounces**	1 **bread, ¹/₂ fat**

*Exchanges based on addition of whole milk

Clam Chowder (New England made with milk)*	10 ounces	1 bread, 1 meat, 1 fat, $^1/_2$ milk
Consomme (Beef)	10 ounces	1 vegetable
Creamy Chicken Mushroom	10 ounces	1 bread, 2 fats
Curly Noodle with Chicken	10 ounces	1 bread, $^1/_2$ fat
Green Pea	11 ounces	2 breads, 1 meat, $^1/_2$ fat
Meatball Alphabet	10 ounces	1 bread, 1 meat, $^1/_2$ fat
Minestrone	10 ounces	1 bread, $^1/_2$ fat
Mushroom, Cream of	10 ounces	1 bread, 1 fat
Mushroom, Golden	10 ounces	1 bread, 1 fat
Noodles & Ground Beef	10 ounces	1 bread, 1 fat
Onion	10 ounces	1 bread, $^1/_2$ fat
Onion, Cream of (made with water and milk)*	10 ounces	1 bread, $^1/_2$ fat, $^1/_2$ milk
Oriental Chicken	10 ounces	1 vegetable, 1 fat
Oyster Stew (made with milk)*	10 ounces	$^1/_2$ bread, $^1/_2$ meat, $1^1/_2$ fats, $^1/_2$ milk
Pepper Pot	10 ounces	1 bread, $^1/_2$ meat, $^1/_2$ fat
Potato, Cream of (made with water and milk)*	10 ounces	1 bread, 1 fat, $^1/_2$ milk
Shrimp, Cream of (made with water and milk)*	10 ounces	1 bread, 2 fats, $^1/_2$ milk
Split Pea with Ham and Bacon	11 ounces	2 breads, 1 meat, $^1/_2$ fat
Tomato	10 ounces	1 vegetable, 1 bread, $^1/_2$ fat
Tomato (made with milk)*	10 ounces	1 vegetable, 1 bread, $1^1/_2$ fats, $^1/_2$ milk
Tomato Bisque	11 ounces	2 breads, $^1/_2$ fat
Tomato Rice, Old Fashioned	11 ounces	2 breads, $^1/_2$ fat
Turkey Noodle	10 ounces	1 bread, $^1/_2$ fat
Turkey Vegetable	10 ounces	1 bread, $^1/_2$ fat
Vegetable	10 ounces	1 vegetable, 1 bread
Vegetable Beef	10 ounces	$^1/_2$ bread, 1 meat
Vegetable, Old Fashioned	10 ounces	1 bread, $^1/_2$ fat
Vegetarian Vegetable	10 ounces	1 bread, $^1/_2$ fat
Won Ton	10 ounces	$^1/_2$ bread, $^1/_2$ meat

CAMPBELL'S SOUP FOR ONE
(All servings 1 can, given in prepared ounces)

Bean, Old Fashioned with Ham	11 ounces	2 breads, $^1/_2$ meat, 1 fat
Burly Vegetable Beef	11 ounces	1 vegetable, 1 bread, 1 meat

Exchanges based on addition of whole milk

Clam Chowder (New England made with whole milk)*	11 ounces	1 bread, ¹/₂ meat, 1¹/₂ fats, ¹/₂ milk
Full Flavored Chicken Vegetable	11 ounces	1 bread, 1 fat
Golden Chicken & Noodles	11 ounces	1 bread, 1 fat
Mushroom, Cream of, savory	11 ounces	1 bread, 2 fats
Tomato Royale	11 ounces	2 breads, 1 fat
Vegetable, Old World	11 ounces	1 bread, 1 fat

CAMPBELL'S CHUNKY SOUPS
(Individual Service Size) 1 can, undiluted oz.

Chunky Beef	10³/₄ ounces	1¹/₂ bread, 1¹/₂ meat
Chunky Beef with Noodles (Stroganoff style)	10³/₄ ounces	2 breads, 1¹/₂ meats, 2 fats
Chunky Chicken	10³/₄ ounces	1¹/₂ breads, 2 meats, ¹/₂ fat
Chunky Chili Beef	11 ounces	2¹/₂ breads, 2¹/₂ meats
Chunky Clam Chowder (Manhattan style)	10³/₄ ounces	1¹/₂ breads, ¹/₂ meat, 1 fat
Chunky Ham 'n Butter Bean	10³/₄ ounces	2 breads, 1¹/₂ meats, 1¹/₂ fats
Chunky Old Fashioned Bean w/Ham	11 ounces	2 breads, 1¹/₂ meats, 1 vegetable, 1¹/₂ fats
Chunky Old Fashioned Vegetable Beef	10³/₄ ounces	1 bread, 1 meat, 1 vegetable, ¹/₂ fat
Chunky Sirloin Burger	10¹/₂ ounces	1 bread, 1¹/₂ meats, 1 vegetable, 1 fat
Chunky Split Pea with Ham	10³/₄ ounces	2 breads, 1 meat, 1 fat
Chunky Steak & Potato	10³/₄ ounces	1¹/₂ breads, 1¹/₂ meats
Chunky Vegetable	10³/₄ ounces	1 bread, 1 vegetable, 1 fat

CAMPBELL'S LOW SODIUM PRODUCTS *(1 can, undiluted oz.)*

Chicken Noodle	7¹/₄ ounces	1 bread, ¹/₂ fat
Chunky Chicken	7¹/₂ ounces	1 bread, 1 meat, ¹/₂ fat
Green Pea	7¹/₂ ounces	1¹/₂ breads, ¹/₂ meat, ¹/₂ fat
Mushroom, Cream of	7¹/₄ ounces	¹/₂ bread, 2 fats
Tomato	7¹/₄ ounces	1 bread, 1 vegetable, 1 fat
Turkey Noodle	7¹/₄ ounces	¹/₂ bread, ¹/₂ fat
Vegetable	7¹/₄ ounces	1 bread, ¹/₂ fat
Vegetable Beef	7¹/₄ ounces	1 vegetable, 1 meat
"V-8" Cocktail Vegetable Juice	6 ounces	1 vegetable

OTHER CAMPBELL CANNED PRODUCTS

Barbecue Beans	4 ounces	1¹/₂ breads, ¹/₂ fat
Home Style Beans	4 ounces	1¹/₂ breads, ¹/₂ fat
Pork & Bean	4 ounces	1¹/₂ breads, ¹/₂ fat
Tomato Juice	6 ounces	1 vegetable

| "V-8" Cocktail Vegetable Juice | 6 ounces | 1 vegetable |
| "V-8" Spicy Hot Cocktail Vegetable Juice | 6 ounces | 1 vegetable |

CAMPBELL'S PASTA

Macaroni with Cheese	1 cup	1$^{1}/_{2}$ breads, 1 meat
Italian Style Spaghetti	1 cup	2 breads
Spaghetti and Ground Beef	1 cup	1$^{1}/_{2}$ breads, 1 meat, 1 fat
Spaghetti and Tomato Sauce	1 cup	2 breads
Spaghetti and Meatballs	1 cup	1$^{1}/_{2}$ breads, 1 meat, 1 fat
Spaghetti Sauce and Meat	1 cup	1 bread, 1 meat, 1 fat
Spaghetti Sauce and Mushrooms	1 cup	1$^{1}/_{2}$ breads, 2 fats

CHEF BOY-AR-DEE PRODUCTS

Spaghetti Sauce with Meat	$^{1}/_{2}$ can (4 ounces)	1 bread, $^{1}/_{2}$ meat, 1 fat
Spaghetti Sauce with Mushrooms	$^{1}/_{2}$ can (4 ounces)	1 bread, $^{1}/_{2}$ meat, 1 fat
Pizza Sauce	2 ounces	1 fat
Mushrooms in Brown Gravy	5 ounces	1 vegetable, 1 fat
Beefaroni	$^{1}/_{3}$ can (5 ounces)	1 bread, 1 meat
Cheese Ravioli	$^{1}/_{3}$ can (5 ounces)	1$^{1}/_{2}$ breads, $^{1}/_{2}$ meat, 1 fat
Chili Con Carne with Beans	$^{1}/_{3}$ can (5 ounces)	1$^{1}/_{2}$ breads, 1 fat
Marinara Sauce	$^{1}/_{2}$ cup	1 bread
Meatballs with Gravy	$^{1}/_{3}$ can (5 ounces)	$^{1}/_{2}$ bread, 2 meat, 1 fat
Ravioli with Beef	$^{1}/_{3}$ can (5 ounces)	1$^{1}/_{2}$ breads, 1 fat
Spaghetti and Meatballs	$^{1}/_{3}$ can (5 ounces)	1 bread, 1 meat
Spaghetti Sauce with Meat	$^{1}/_{3}$ can (5 ounces)	1 bread, 1 fat
Spaghetti Sauce with Meatballs	$^{1}/_{3}$ can (5 ounces)	1$^{1}/_{2}$ breads, 1 meat, 1 fat
Spaghetti Sauce with Mushrooms	$^{1}/_{3}$ can (5 ounces)	1 bread, $^{1}/_{2}$ fat
Meatball Stew	$^{1}/_{4}$ can (7 ounces)	1 bread, 1 meat, 1 fat
Lasagna	$^{1}/_{5}$ can (8 ounces)	2$^{1}/_{2}$ breads, 1 fat
Ravioli with Beef	$^{1}/_{5}$ can (8 ounces)	2$^{1}/_{2}$ breads, 1 fat
Spaghetti & Meatballs	$^{1}/_{5}$ can (8 ounces)	2 breads, 1 meat, $^{1}/_{2}$ fat
Pizza Pie Mix (made with water)	$^{1}/_{4}$	2 breads, 1 fat
Spaghetti & Meatball Dinner	$^{1}/_{6}$	3 bread, 1 meat
Spaghetti with Meat Dinner	$^{1}/_{6}$	2$^{1}/_{2}$ breads, 1 meat
Spaghetti with Mushroom Dinner	$^{1}/_{6}$	2$^{1}/_{2}$ breads

Pizza with Sausage	$^1/_6$	1$^1/_2$ breads, $^1/_2$ meat, 1 fat
Frozen Beef Ravioli	$^1/_2$ can (8 ounces)	2$^1/_2$ breads, 1 meat, 1 fat
Frozen Cheese Ravioli	$^1/_2$ can (8 ounces)	2 breads, 1 meat, 1 fat
Frozen Lasagna	$^1/_2$ can (8 ounces)	1$^1/_2$ breads, 2 meats, 1 fat
Frozen Manicotti	$^1/_2$ can (8 ounces)	2 breads, 2 meats, 3 fats

CHUN KING CORP.

Chicken Chow Mein, divider-pak	$^1/_4$ total mix	2 breads, 2 meats
Beef Chow Mein, divider-pak	$^1/_4$ total mix	2 breads, 2 meats, 1 fat
Mushroom Chow Mein, divider-pak	$^1/_4$ total mix	2 breads
Meatless Chow Mein	$^1/_2$ can	1 bread
Subgum Chicken Chow Mein	$^1/_2$ can	1 bread
Beef Chop Suey	$^1/_2$ can	1 bread
Chinese Vegetables	$^1/_2$ can	Free Food
Chop Suey Vegetables	$^1/_2$ can	Free Food
Bean Sprouts	$^1/_2$ can	Free Food
Chow Mein Noodles	$^1/_2$ can	$^1/_2$ breads, 2 fats
Frozen Chicken Chow Mein	$^1/_2$ pkg. (8 ounces)	1 bread, 1 meat
Soy Sauce	—	Free Food

FRANCO-AMERICAN PRODUCTS *(Serving size in ounces)*

Beef Ravioli in Meat Sauce	7$^1/_2$ ounces	2 breads, 1 vegetable, 1 meat
Beef RavioliO's in Meat Sauce	7$^1/_2$ ounces	Same
BeefyO's (O-shaped macaroni and beef in tomato sauce)	7$^1/_2$ ounces	1$^1/_2$ breads, 1 meat, 1 fat, 1 vegetable
CheeseO's (O-shaped macaroni in tangy cheese sauce)	7$^1/_2$ ounces	1$^1/_2$ breads, 1 meat, $^1/_2$ fat
Cheese RavioliO's in tomato sauce	7$^1/_2$ ounces	2 breads, $^1/_2$ meat, 1$^1/_2$ fats, 1 vegetable
Elbow Macaroni & Cheese	7$^3/_8$ ounces	1$^1/_2$ breads, $^1/_2$ meat, 1 fat
Macaroni & Cheese	7$^3/_8$ ounces	1$^1/_2$ breads, $^1/_2$ meat, 1 fat
PizzaO's (O-shaped macaroni in zesty pizza sauce)	7$^1/_2$ ounces	2 breads, 1 vegetable
Spaghetti in Meat Sauce	7$^1/_2$ ounces	1 bread, 1 meat, 1$^1/_2$ fats, 1 vegetable
Spaghetti in Tomato Sauce with Cheese	7$^3/_8$ ounces	2 breads, 1 vegetable
Spaghetti with Meatballs in Tomato Sauce	7$^3/_8$ ounces	1 bread, 1 meat, 1 fat, 1 vegetable
SpaghettiO's in Tomato and Cheese Sauce	7$^3/_8$ ounces	2 breads, 1 vegetable

GOLDEN GRAIN CO.

Spaghetti Dinner	1 cup	3 breads, 1 fat
Cheese Rice-A-Roni	1 cup	2¹/₂ breads, 1 meat, 1 fat
Spanish Rice-A-Roni	1 cup	2¹/₂ breads, 2 fats
Wild Rice-A-Roni	1 cup	3 breads, 2 fats
Twist-A-Roni	1 cup	2¹/₂ breads, 1 fat
Scallop-A-Roni	1 cup	2 breads, 1 meat

GREEN GIANT

Broccoli-Cauliflower Medley	¹/₂ cup	¹/₂ bread, ¹/₂ vegetable, ¹/₂ fat
Broccoli Fanfare	¹/₂ cup	¹/₂ bread, 1 vegegable, ¹/₂ fat
Cauliflower in Cheese Sauce	¹/₂ cup	1 vegetable, ¹/₂ fat
Okra Gumbo	¹/₂ cup	1 vegetable, 2 fats
Rice and Broccoli	¹/₂ cup	1 vegetable, 1 bread, 1 fat
Rice with Peas and Mushrooms	¹/₂ cup	1 vegetable, 1 bread, ¹/₂ fat
Rice Pilaf	¹/₂ cup	1¹/₂ breads, ¹/₂ fat
White and Wild Rice	¹/₂ cup	1¹/₂ breads, ¹/₂ fat

KRAFT A LA CARTE SINGLE SERVING POUCHES

Beef Stew	one pouch	2 meats, 1¹/₂ breads, 2¹/₂ fats
Macaroni and Beef	one pouch	2 meats, 1¹/₂ breads, 1¹/₂ fats
Salisbury Steak	one pouch	2 meats, ¹/₂ bread, 1¹/₂ fats
Sweet 'n Sour Pork	one pouch	2 meats, 2 breads, 1 fat

KRAFT MIXES

American-style Spaghetti Dinner Mix	1 cup	3 breads, 1 fat
Cheese Pizza Mix	¹/₄ box	1 meat, 2¹/₂ breads, 1 fat
Macaroni and Cheese Dinner Mix	1 cup	¹/₂ meat, 2¹/₂ breads, 1¹/₂ fats

MORTON BRAND TV DINNERS

Ham	1 package	1 bread, 5 meat (omit applesauce)
Turkey, Beef, Salisbury Steak, Meatloaf, and Fish	1 package	1 bread, 1 vegetable, 5 meats
Shrimp	1 package	1 bread, 1 vegetable, 4 meats, 1 fat

RAGU BRAND

Homestyle Spaghetti Sauce	4 ounce serving	1 bread, ¹/₂ fat
Homestyle Spaghetti Sauce with Mushrooms	4 ounce serving	1 bread, ¹/₂ fat

Homestyle Spaghetti Sauce flavored with Meat	4 ounce serving	1 bread, ¹/₂ fat

SWANSON CANNED PRODUCTS

Chunk Chicken	2¹/₂ ounces	2 meats
Chunk White Chicken	2¹/₂ ounces	2 meats
Chunk Thigh Chicken	2¹/₂ ounces	2 meats
Chunk Style Mixin Chicken	2¹/₂ ounces	2 meats, ¹/₂ fat
Chunk Turkey	2¹/₂ ounces	2 meats
Chicken Spread	1 ounce	¹/₂ meat, 1 fat
Beef Broth	7¹/₄ ounces	Free Food (18 calorie serving)
Chicken Broth	7¹/₄ ounces	1 fat
Beef Stew	7⁵/₈ ounces	1 bread, 1 meat, ¹/₂ fat
Chicken Stew	7⁵/₈ ounces	1 bread, 1 meat, 1 fat
Chicken a la King	5¹/₄ ounces	¹/₂ bread, 1 meat, 2 fats
Chicken and Dumplings	7¹/₂ ounces	1 bread, 1 meat, 2 fats

SWANSON FROZEN PRODUCTS (MEAT PIES)

Beef	one 8 ounce pie	3 breads, 1 meat, 4 fats
Chicken	one 8 ounce pie	3 breads, 1 meat, 4 fats
Turkey	one 8 ounce pie	3 breads, 1 meat, 4¹/₂ fats
Macaroni and Cheese	one 7 ounce pie	2 breads, 1 meat, 1 fat

SWANSON FROZEN HUNGRY-MAN MEAT PIES

Beef	one 16 ounce pie	4 breads, 3 meats, 7 fats, 1 vegetable
Chicken	one 16 ounce pie	same as beef
Steakburger	one 16 ounce pie	4 breads, 3 meats, 8 fats, 1 vegetable
Turkey	one 16 ounce pie	4 breads, 3 meats, 7¹/₂ fats, 1 vegetable

SWANSON FROZEN ENTREES *(one complete entree, Oz.)*

Chicken Nibbles with French Fries	5 ounces	2 breads, 1¹/₂ meats, 3 fats
Fish 'n Chips	5 ounces	1¹/₂ breads, 2 meats, 2 fats
French Toast with Sausages	4¹/₂ ounces	1¹/₂ breads, 2 meats, 2 fats
Fried Chicken with Whipped Potatoes	7¹/₄ ounces	2 breads, 2¹/₂ meats, 3 fats
Gravy and Sliced Beef with Whipped Potatoes	8 ounces	1 bread, 2 meats, ¹/₂ fat
Meatballs with Brown Gravy and Whipped Potatoes	9¹/₄ ounces	2 breads, 2 meats, 2 fats
Meatloaf with Tomato Sauce and Whipped Potatoes	9 ounces	2 breads, 2 meats, 2 fats

Omelets with Cheese Sauce and Ham	8 ounces	1 bread, 2¹/₂ meats, 4 fats
Pancakes and Sausages	6 ounces	3 breads, 1 meat, 5 fats
Salisbury Steak w/Crinkle-Cut Potatoes	5¹/₂ ounces	2 breads, 1¹/₂ meats, 3 fats
Scrambled Eggs and Sausage with Hash Brown Potatoes	6¹/₄ ounces	1¹/₂ breads, 2 meats, 5 fats
Spaghetti with Breaded Veal	8¹/₄ ounces	1¹/₂ breads, 1 meat, 2 fats, 1 vegetable
Spanish Style Omelet	8 ounces	1 bread, 1 meat, 3 fats
Turkey/Gravy/Dressing with Whipped Potatoes	8³/₄ ounces	1¹/₂ breads, 2 meats, 1 fat

SWANSON HUNGRY MAN ENTREES

Barbecue Flavored Chicken with Whipped Potatoes	12 ounces*	3 breads, 4 meats, 3 fats
Fried Chicken with Whipped Potatoes	12 ounces*	2¹/₂ breads, 5 meats, 4 fats
Fried Chicken Breast Portions	11³/₄ ounces*	3 breads, 6 meats, 4 fats
Fried Chicken Drumsticks	10³/₄ ounces*	2¹/₂ breads, 4 meats, 5 fats
Lasagna and Garlic Roll	12³/₄ ounces	3 breads, 2 meats, 5 fats
Salisbury Steak w/Crinkle-Cut Potatoes	12¹/₂ ounces	2¹/₂ breads, 4 meats, 5¹/₂ fats
Sliced Beef with Whipped Potatoes	12¹/₄ ounces	1¹/₂ breads, 4 meats
Turkey/Gravy/Dressing with Whipped Potatoes	13¹/₄ ounces	2 breads, 4 meats, ¹/₂ fat

SWANSON FROZEN MAIN COURSE *(One complete entree, Oz.)*

Chicken Cacciatore	11¹/₂ ounces	¹/₂ bread, 4 meats, 1 vegetable
Chicken in White Wine Sauce	8¹/₄ ounces	1 bread, 3 meats, 3 fats
Creamed Chipped Beef	10¹/₂ ounces	1 bread, 2 meats, 3¹/₂ fats
Filet of Haddock Almondine	7¹/₂ ounces	¹/₂ bread, 4 meats, 2¹/₂ fats
Lasagna with Meat in Tomato Sauce	12¹/₄ ounces	3¹/₂ breads, 2 meats, 3 fats
Macaroni and Cheese	12 ounces	2¹/₂ breads, 2 meats, 3 fats
Salisbury Steak with Gravy	10 ounces	1 bread, 3¹/₂ meats, 3¹/₂ fats
Steak and Green Peppers in Oriental Style Sauce	8¹/₂ ounces	¹/₂ bread, 2¹/₂ meats, 1 vegetable
Turkey with Gravy and Dressing	9¹/₄ ounces	1¹/₂ breads, 4 meats

Exchanges based on addition of whole milk

CARBOHYDRATE CONTENT OF VARIOUS
BRAND NAME CEREALS

Each of the cereals listed below has the calories given in terms of how much is in one ounce of cereal. A helping of cereal is always noted in terms of how much carbohydrate is in one ounce, except for raisin bran cereals. Those cereals with raisins are understood to have one ounce of cereal and 3/10 ounce of raisins per helping. Starches and related complex carbohydrates are in one category, and sucrose (table sugar) and other sugars are listed in a second category. Amounts are listed in grams. The amount of fiber, if any, is also listed, followed by the total amount of carbohydrate. Most fiber is understood to be indigestible and, therefore, has no intrinsic food value. To get the total grams of carbohydrate if 1/2 cup (4 oz.) of skim milk is consumed with the cereal portion, add another 6 grams of carbohydrate.

Each helping of cereal is assumed to have this 1/2 cup of skim milk added to it, making the total carbohydrate content increase by about 6 grams, as mentioned above. This last bit of carbohydrate comes from the milk sugar, or lactose content, of the skim milk.

NAME OF CEREAL	STARCH AND RELATED	SUCROSE AND OTHER SUGARS	FIBER	TOTAL
Buc Wheats	15	9	–	24
Cheerios	19	1	–	20
Cocoa Puffs	14	11	–	25
Count Chocula	11	13	–	24
Crispy Wheats 'n Raisins	13	10	–	23
Golden Grahams	14	10	–	24
Honey Nut Cheerios	13	10	–	23
Kaboom	17	6	–	23
Kix	22	2	–	24
Lucky Charms	13	11	–	24
Powdered Donutz	12	10	–	22
Raisin Nut Bran	11	7	3	21
Rocky Road	10	13	–	23
S'Mores Crunch	14	10	–	24
KELLOGG'S CEREALS				
All Bran	7	5	9	27
All Bran Fruit & Almonds	9	9	10	28

DUTCH DIET

Apple Jacks	12	14	–	26
Banana Frosted Flakes	15	10	–	25
Cocoa Krispies	13	12	–	25
Corn Flakes	23	2	–	25
Crackling Bran	8	8	4	20
40% Bran Flakes	14	5	4	23
Frosted Mini Wheats	15	7	2	24
Frosted Rice Krispies	15	11	–	26
Fruit Loops	12	13	–	25
Fruitful Bran	15	11	4	30
Graham Crackos	14	10	–	24
Honey & Nut Corn Flakes	15	9	–	24
Just Right	22	6	2	30
Most	12	6	4	22
Nutrigrain Wheat	20	2	2	24
Nutrigrain Wheat & Raisins	22	8	2	32
Product 19	21	3	–	24
Raisin Bran	12	12	4	28
Raisin & Rice	21	10	–	31
Raisin Squares	14	5	3	22
Rice & Rye	21	10	–	31
Rice Krispies	22	3	–	25
Special K	19	2	–	21
Sugar Corn Pops	14	12	–	26
Sugar Frosted Flakes	15	11	–	26
Sugar Smacks	9	16	–	25

NABISCO CEREALS

100% BRAN	6	6	9	21
Shredded Wheat (No sugar or salt added) 1 biscuit	19	–	–	19
Shredded Wheat, Spoon Size	23	–	–	23
Team	19	5	–	24

NATURE VALLEY

Granola with Fruit & Nuts	12	8	–	20

POST CEREALS

Fruit and Fibre:				
Dates Raisins Walnuts	11	7	4	22
Harvest Medley	11	7	4	22
Mountain Trail	11	7	4	22
Tropical Fruit	12	6	4	22
New Horizon Trail Mix	14	8	–	22
100% Natural Cereal	11	6	–	17
100% Natural Cereal with Raisins & Dates	13	5	–	18

RALSTON PURINA CEREALS

Bran Chex	13	5	5	23
Cookie Crisp	12	13	–	25

Corn Chex	23	2	–	25
Rice Chex	23	2	–	25
Sun Flakes with Nutrasweet	24	–	–	24
Waffelo's, Blueberry	12	13	–	25
Waffelo's, Maple	12	13	–	25
Wheat Chex	19	2	2	23

Beware of the numbers of "natural" granola-type cereals that are loaded with sugars, honey, corn syrup, and other high density nutrients. These "natural" cereals will help you put on lots of "natural" fat where you don't want it. If you want a real natural cereal, consider regular, unflavored oatmeal. This type of cereal of the Quaker Oats type is one of the best sources of fiber, minerals, and other nutrients found in oats. It is probably best to stay away from the instant type of oatmeal that is flavored with one or another extra ingredient. These ingredients may be too high in sugars. Become a label reader. All of the information listed above, plus that for cereals I didn't list, is available for you on the packages of most name brands. If a package doesn't have this information, refuse to buy it. All of the major manufacturers do you the courtesy of listing this information. Buy only when you're SURE of what you're buying.

FROZEN DINNERS WITH 300 CALORIES OR LESS

Each of the food manufacturers listed in this section has put together a group of convenience foods that can be rapidly defrosted and cooked in an oven or microwave. At the time this book was written, all of the exchange (portion) information had not been made available to me for use by you. However, each company has a consumer products division with the address printed on the individual carton of each entree.

The best way to deal with the problem of calculating how these entrees fit into your daily food calculations is to pick either the calorie count or the type of portion count (e.g., 2 lean meat portions and 1½ bread portions) which is printed on the carton or available from the manufacturer. Whatever the case, deduct that amount from your daily food intake allowance.

Where there are portion counts listed, just omit the number of portions in each category of food. If only the calorie count is listed, deduct that from your daily intake and step down to the next lowest calorie chart for the remainder of your food for that day. This second way of handling things is a little inexact, but close enough for everyone except diabetics on insulin.

One example might be Benihana's Chicken in Spicy Garlic Sauce, with a calorie count of 280. You are allowed 1,500 calories for the entire day. Omit three hundred calories, giving you a remainder of 1,200 calories for the rest of your meals that day. Instead of using the 1,500 calorie chart, use the 1,200 calorie chart and add the 300 calorie entree.

If the entree has less than 300 calories, but more than 260, simply deduct the 300 from the total. If there are from 220 to 260 calories, deduct 300 calories from the total daily calories (to account for a convenience entree), and add an extra fruit or cooked vegetable portion to the daily food ration. If there are from 180 to 220 calories in the entree, deduct 300 calories for the entree, plus add one extra bread and one extra fruit to the daily intake. This is not as complicated as it seems, and you will soon get used to these calculations.

ENTREE NAME	NUMBER OF CALORIES	GRAMS OF PROTEIN	GRAMS OF CARBOHYDRATE	GRAMS OF FAT
BENIHANA FROZEN FOOD CORPORATION				
Chicken & Pineapple	280	17	45	4
Chicken in Spicy Garlic Sauce	280	20	43	4
Oriental Style Shrimp with Rice	250	12	42	4
Oriental Glazed Chicken	240	20	34	3
Roast Pork and Mushrooms	260	16	35	7
Seafood Supreme	260	13	40	6
Shrimp in Spicy Garlic Sauce	240	13	41	3
CANDLE LITE ENTREES — WEIGHT WATCHERS INTERNATIONAL				
Beef Sirloin Tips	260	27	21	8
Beef Teriyaki	300	23	31	9
Chicken Cordon Bleu	330	21	31	13

Sweet & Sour				
Pork	270	20	28	9

CLASSIC LITE (ARMOUR FOOD COMPANY)

Beef Pepper Steak	270	21	27	9
Chicken				
Burgundy	230	24	25	4
Chicken Oriental	250	24	26	6
Medallions of				
Chicken Breast				
Marsala	270	22	28	7
Seafood in				
Natural herbs	250	12	38	6
Turf N Surf	250	31	14	7

DINING LITE (BLUE STARS FOOD INC.)

Chicken a la King				
with Rice	290	16	38	7
Glazed Chicken				
with Vegetable				
Rice	250	23	29	4
Lasagna (Cheese				
& Vegetables)	270	19	39	4
Oriental Pepper				
Steak & Rice	290	19	38	6
Spaghetti with				
Beef &				
Mushroom				
Sauce	280	18	41	4

LIGHT AND ELEGANT FOODS

Beef Stroganoff &				
Parsley Noodles	260	24	27	6
Chicken in				
Cheese Sauce	290	19	30	11
Lasagna				
Florentine	280	24	34	5
Macaroni &				
Cheese	300	15	37	9
Shrimp Creole,				
Rice, Peppers	200	11	31	2
Sliced Turkey &				
Gravy	230	20	25	5
Spaghetti with				
Meat Sauce	290	16	40	8

LEAN CUISINE

Each entree listed here has a number of figures representing its nutritional composition. After the name I have listed the number of calories and the American Dietetic Association exchanges present per entree. Meat portions are either shown to be MF(medium-fat) or L (low-fat) in type. All entrees contain one serving per container.

ENTREE NAME	NUMBER OF CALORIES	ADA EXCHANGES
Beef and pork canneloni, Mornay sauce	260	1¹/₂ MF, 1 starch, ¹/₂ veg, ¹/₂ milk
Beefsteak Ranchero	270	1¹/₂ L, 1¹/₂ starch, 1 veg, 1 fat
Breast of chicken in herb cream sauce	260	2¹/₂ L, ¹/₂ starch, ¹/₂ veg, ¹/₂ milk
Breast of chicken Marsala, vegetables	190	2¹/₂ L, ¹/₂ starch, 1 veg
Breast of chicken Parmesan	250	2¹/₂ L, 1 starch, 1 veg
Cheese cannelloni, tomato sauce	260	2 L, 1 starch, 1 veg
Chicken a l'orange, almond rice	260	2 L, 2 starch
Chicken & vegetables, vermicelli	270	2 L, 1¹/₂ starch, 1 veg, ¹/₂ fat
Chicken cacciatore, vermicelli	270	2¹/₂ L, 1 starch, 2 veg
Chicken chow mein, rice	250	1 L, 2 starch, 1 veg
Chicken Oriental	240	2 L, 1¹/₂ starch, ¹/₂ veg
Filet of fish Divan	260	3 L, ¹/₂ starch, ¹/₂ veg, ¹/₂ milk
Filet of fish Florentine	240	3L, 1 veg, ¹/₂ milk
Filet of fish jardiniere, souffled potatoes	280	3L, ¹/₂ starch, 1 veg, ¹/₂ milk
Glazed chicken, vegetable rice	270	3L, 1¹/₂ starch
Lasagna, meat & sauce	270	2¹/₂ L, 1¹/₂ starch, ¹/₂ veg
Linguini, clam sauce	260	1¹/₂ L, 2 starch, ¹/₂ fat
Meatball stew	250	2¹/₂ L, 1 starch, ¹/₂ veg, ¹/₂ fat
Oriental beef, vegetables, rice	250	2 L, 1¹/₂ starch, ¹/₂ veg
Rigatoni bake, meat sauce, cheese	260	2 MF, 1 starch, 1¹/₂ veg
Salisbury steak, Italian sauce, vegetables	280	3 L, ¹/₂ starch, 1 veg, 1 fat
Shrimp & chicken Cantonese, noodles	260	2¹/₂ L, 1 starch, 1 veg, ¹/₂ fat
Sliced turkey breast, mushroom sauce	240	2 L, 1 starch, ¹/₂ veg, ¹/₂ milk
Spaghetti, beef and mushroom sauce	280	1 MF, 2 starch, 1¹/₂ veg
Stuffed cabbage, meat and tomato sauce	220	1¹/₂ MF, ¹/₂ starch, 2 veg, ¹/₂ fat
Szechwan beef, noodles and vegetables	260	2 L, 1¹/₂ starch, ¹/₂ veg, ¹/₂ fat
Tuna lasagna, spinach noodles and vegetables	270	1¹/₂ MF, 1 starch, ¹/₂ veg, ¹/₂ milk, ¹/₂ fat
Turkey Dijon	270	2¹/₂ L, ¹/₂ starch, 1 veg, ¹/₂ milk, ¹/₂ fat
Veal primavera	250	2¹/₂ L, 1 starch, ¹/₂ veg, ¹/₂ fat

Vegetables and pasta Mornay with ham	280	1 MF, 1 starch, 1 veg, $\frac{1}{2}$ milk, 1 fat
Zucchini lasagna	260	2 L, $1\frac{1}{2}$ starch, 1 veg

WEIGHT WATCHERS FROZEN ENTREES

Weight Watchers portion designations are slightly different from the ADA ones, but close enough for you to get a good idea about their nutritional composition. Each entree is a single serving.

ENTREE NAME	CALORIES	PORTION CONTENT
Chicken fettucini	290	2 protein, $1\frac{1}{2}$ starch, 1 fat, $\frac{1}{4}$ milk, 10 optional calories
Stuffed turkey breast	270	2 protein, $\frac{1}{2}$ starch, 1 fat, $1\frac{1}{2}$ veg, 10 optional calories
Southern fried chicken patty	270	3 protein, 1 starch, $\frac{1}{2}$ veg, 2 fats
Chicken nuggets	180	2 protein, $\frac{1}{2}$ starch, 1 fat
Chicken patty parmigiana	280	3 protein, $\frac{1}{2}$ starch, 1 fat, $1\frac{1}{2}$ veg
Imperial chicken	230	2 protein, 1 starch, 1 veg, $\frac{1}{2}$ fat, 10 optional calories
Chicken ala king	230	2 protein, $\frac{1}{2}$ starch, $\frac{1}{2}$ veg, 1 fat, $\frac{1}{2}$ milk, 10 optional calories
Sweet 'n sour chicken tenders	250	$1\frac{1}{2}$ protein, 1 starch, 1 veg, 1 fruit, 10 optional calories
Beef Salisbury steak Romana	320	$2\frac{1}{2}$ protein, 1 starch, 1 veg, 1 fat
Chopped beef steak	280	3 protein, 1 veg, 10 optional calories
Veal patty parmigiana	240	3 protein, $1\frac{1}{2}$ veg
Beef Stroganoff	340	2 protein, 1 starch, $\frac{1}{2}$ veg, 1 fat, $\frac{1}{4}$ milk, 10 optional calories
Filet of fish au gratin	210	$3\frac{1}{2}$ protein, $\frac{1}{2}$ starch, 1 veg, 10 optional calories
Oven fried fish	220	3 protein, $\frac{1}{2}$ starch, $\frac{1}{2}$ veg, 2 fat
Stuffed sole with newburg sauce	310	$2\frac{1}{2}$ protein, 1 starch, $\frac{1}{2}$ veg, 1 fat, $\frac{1}{2}$ milk, 10 optional calories
Seafood linguini	220	$1\frac{1}{2}$ protein, 1 starch, $\frac{1}{2}$ veg, 1 fat, 5 optional calories
Broccoli and cheese baked potato	280	1 protein, $1\frac{1}{2}$ starch, 1 veg, $\frac{1}{4}$ milk, 5 optional calories
Chicken divan baked potato	290	$1\frac{1}{2}$ protein, $1\frac{1}{2}$ starch, $\frac{1}{2}$ veg, $\frac{1}{4}$ milk, 10 optional calories

Pasta Primavera	290	1 protein, 1 starch, 1 veg, $^1/_2$ fat, $^1/_4$ milk, 10 optional calories
Lasagna with meat sauce	340	2 protein, 1 starch, 1 veg, $^1/_2$ fat, 10 optional calories
Italian cheese lasagna	370	2 protein, 1 starch, 1 veg, $^1/_2$ fat, 10 optional calories
Pasta rigati	290	2 protein, 1 starch, 1 veg, 10 optional calories
Baked cheese ravioli	310	2 protein, 1 starch,1 veg, 5 optional calories
Spaghetti with meat sauce	280	$1^1/_2$ protein, $1^1/_2$ starch, 1 veg, $^1/_2$ fat
Cheese manicotti	290	2 protein, 1 starch, 1 veg, $^1/_2$ fat, 10 optional calories
Chicken fajitas	260	$1^1/_2$ protein, $1^1/_2$ starch, 1 veg, 10 optional calories
Beef fajitas	270	$1^1/_2$ protein, $1^1/_2$ starch, 1 veg, 5 optional calories
Chicken enchiladas Suiza	360	2 protein, 1 starch, $^1/_2$ veg, $^1/_4$ milk, 10 optional calories
Beef enchiladas ranchero	310	2 protein, 1 starch, 1 veg, 10 optional calories
Cheese enchiladas ranchero	370	2 protein, 1 starch, 1 veg, 10 optional calories
Beefsteak burrito	330	$1^1/_2$ protein, $1^1/_2$ starch, 1 veg, $^1/_2$ fat, 20 optional calories
Chicken burrito	330	$1^1/_2$ protein, $1^1/_2$ starch, 1 veg, 1 fat, 20 optional calories
Deluxe combination pizza	290	$1^1/_2$ protein, $1^1/_2$ starch, $^1/_2$ veg, 10 optional calories
Sausage pizza	310	2 protein, $1^1/_2$ starch, $^1/_4$ veg
Pepperoni pizza	320	$1^1/_2$ protein, $1^1/_2$ starch, $^1/_4$ veg
Cheese pizza	320	2 protein, 2 starch, $^1/_4$ veg
Pepperoni French bread pizza	330	$1^1/_2$ protein, 2 starch, 1 fat, $^1/_2$ veg
Cheese French bread pizza	320	$1^1/_2$ protein, 2 starch, 1 fat, $^1/_2$ veg
Deluxe French bread pizza	330	$1^1/_2$ protein, 2 starch, $^1/_2$ fat, $^1/_2$ veg, 10 optional calories

The vegetable portion in a lot of the above, particularly the Italian style dishes, comes from tomato paste.

APPENDIX ONE

THE COOPER CHART SYSTEM FOR PORTION CONTROL

The instructions in the Dutch Diet book make reference to a system of color-coded designations for use in learning about, and keeping up with, the portions of each type of food used in weight reduction, or in maintenance of an ideal weight, once that goal is reached.

There is an address and phone number given below that will allow you to get these charts and the easy to use learning system that goes with them. These special charts are small enough to be carried in pocket or purse and represent just about every kind of usable food or beverage found on a diet. You may also order the type of vitamin recommended in this book from the same people, unless you have a similar one obtainable locally.

There are seven different color-coded categories, as mentioned in this book, each representing a different category of food. Each measured amount of food listed on the charts is equivalent in calories and nutritional content (fats, protein, carbohydrates) to all the others of that same category and color-coding. Food choices may be substituted or interchanged freely, as long as they are in the same group and of the same color-coding. Sometimes only a half-portion is used at one time, so I have taken that into account with half-portion spaces on the charts.

The food portions can be moved to any part of the day, including snack times and bedtime eating. As long as you "spend" your calories by the end of the day, it doesn't matter when you have them.

DUTCH DIET

A person would use the food tables from the accompanying instruction booklet that comes with the charts, or the more abbreviated tables on the charts themselves, to get quantities of a food portion group for each meal or snack.

You count up all of your allotted portions of each type for the level of calorie intake you are at for the day and write them into the spaces provided on the charts. As you use your portions during the day, you note down on the charts what you have had so far for that day. At the end of the day all the portions allotted from each food group should have been consumed and noted in the appropriate columns.

Think of these portions as if they were money. You have so much to spend and when those are gone, there are no more. If you run out of a particular category, there are no credit cards to use from tomorrow's allotment. You also can't substitute one category of portion for another. If you run out of fruit but still have milk left, you are not allowed to substitute a "white" food for an "orange" one. This system can convert an exchange diet from an overwhelming and complex job into its simplest terms. A dieter can feel free to write food portion sizes on the different places on the chart if something that is preferred isn't on the lists but is in his or her diet plan. By being resourceful and innovative, a lot of foods can be included and accounted for in a diet plan.

This chart system has been tested and found to be effective in teaching a sometimes difficult food accounting task to those persons who need it badly, either for weight loss, or for diabetic portion control. If you wish to order these useful charts, either for yourself or for a friend who is overweight, diabetic, or must follow his or her food intake carefully, call or write Greentree Press at the phone number or address given below.

Greentree Press, Department M.; 3603 West 12th Street, Erie, PA 16505. Phone for faster service is 1-814-833-6353.

APPENDIX TWO

LIST OF SUPPLIERS

I have tried not to endorse or recommend many things that might be required for you while on this diet program, but when I include too few, I get a lot of phone calls from patients who object to the sparcity of information. The names and addresses and phone numbers of suppliers listed below are not the only possible sources for a number of these items. They are the ones I use and trust, but you may have others equally good.

MALSOVIT BREAD AND MEALWAFERS

For information on the baker closest to you who carries Malsovit products, call 1-800-521-3505. They also can supply you by mail if you are temporarily unable to get Malsovit locally.

VITAMIN SUPPLEMENTS

My primary recommendation is the formula detailed in Chapter Six of this book. If you have problems getting this specific one, you may order the vitamins directly from Greentree Press (address and phone given on the previous page), a reputable mail order house that sells books and health-related products.

Food Scales

There are a lot of scales being sold for dieters, but my favorite is the Skinny Scale, sold by IDL Corporation, 730 Garden Street, Carlstadt, NJ 07072. They come in several sizes and are reasonable in price.

Fitness Master

The Fitness Master line of aerobic equipment is sold by the company of the same name. You may contact them for further information at 1-800-328-8995. The unit I use is the Sierra.

Walden Farms Salad Dressings

These salad dressings are tasty and convenient to use, with both bottles and individual packs available in a number of flavors. Call or write them at: Walden Farms, P.O. Box 352, Linden, NJ 07036, 1-201-925-9494. They can either supply you by mail, or let you know of a local bariatric medicine specialist or store that carries their brand.

Thompson Kitchens

This is a company that carries the BatterLite-Whitlock brands of dietary foods that I often recommend. For information about their company and how you may buy their products locally, or by mail order, call 1-800-458-5719. At this time, they also carry the Pritikin line of salad dressings.

APPENDIX THREE

RECIPES FOR SLIMMERS

The recipes given in this appendix are courtesy of members of the Calorie Control Council, Suite 500-D, 5775 Peachtree-Dunwoody Road, Atlanta, Georgia 30342. A list of recipe sources is included at the end of this chapter, but the source of each recipe is also listed following the name. You are encouraged to write these companies for further information about their products if desired.

Where possible, I have grouped these recipes into categories and have included as much about their nutritional equivalents as I have gotten from the authors, or my own calculations. When calculating how to figure them into the Dutch Diet, subtract whatever a serving has in the different food groups from your daily intake. An example would be the Peach Ginger Froth. A serving is eight ounces, with an equivalent food value content of $^1/_2$ nonfat milk portion and $^1/_2$ fruit portion per serving. You would then give up $^1/_2$ portion of each and deduct that from your intake for the day.

As a convention for abbreviations, GDS stands for G.D. Searle, as well as NutraSweet Consumer Products. SB stands for Shasta Beverages. CPC means the Cumberland Packing Corp., makers of the different Sweet'n Low products. For more than one serving, multiply the amount of ingredients by the number of servings.

COLD OR HOT LIQUID TREATS

Strawberry Lemon Spritz — GDS

A fizzy and flavorful alternative to traditional lemonade. Great after an exercise session.

Ingredients One Serving

Fresh or unsweetened frozen strawberries	1 cup
Club soda	1/2 cup
Lemon juice	2 tablespoons (tbl)
Equal	1-2 packets

Puree strawberries in blender. Combine all ingredients in tall glass. Stir well. Add enough ice to fill glass. 44 calories per 8-ounce serving, 1 fruit.

Dublin Cream Cordial — GDS

All the rich, smooth taste of the famous Irish cream cordial, but without the alcohol. Serve straight up or over ice

Ingredients Eight Servings

1 cup nonfat dry milk powder	1/4 tsp brandy extract
1/2 cup warm water	1/8 tsp almond extract
2 tsp instant coffee crystals	2 eggs
or 1/2 tsp unsweetened cocoa powder	2 cups skim milk
powder (decaffeinated if desired)	1 tsp vanilla extract
24 packets Equal	

Combine first 4 ingredients in blender. Blend on high for 50-10 minutes, or until thick and creamy. Add extracts, cocoa and eggs. Blend until well-mixed. Add milk and blend until smooth and creamy. Refrigerate until chilled. Pour into cordial glasses. Best used within 4 days. Makes 8 servings of 4 ounces each, with 110 calories per serving, 1 non-fat milk each.

Strawberry Chocolate Shake — GDS

Ingredients One Serving

Fresh or unsweetened frozen strawberries	1/2 cup
Skim milk	1/2 cup
Unsweetened cocoa powder	2 tsp
Equal	2-3 packets

Combine all ingredients in blender. (Add 3-4 ice cubes if using fresh strawberries.) Blend on high for 30 seconds or until smooth and creamy. Pour into tall glass and serve with straw. 93 calories per 10-ounce serving, 1/2 nonfat milk and 1 fruit.

Banana Chocolate Shake — GDS

Follow strawberry chocolate shake recipe, but substitute 1 medium banana for the strawberries. About the same calories and portion amounts.

Chocolate Amaretto Creme — GDS

Ingredients One Serving

Evaporated skim milk	1/3 cup
Club soda	1/4 cup
Unsweetened cocoa powder	1/2 tbl
Equal	2-3 packets
Almond extract	1/4 tsp
Bitters	1 dash
Ice	1-2 cubes

Combine all ingredients in blender. Blend on high for 10 seconds, or until smooth and creamy. Pour into cocktail glass and serve with straw. 87 calories per 6-ounce serving, 1 nonfat milk.

Chablis Spritzer — GDS

Garnish with Equal-frosted grapes on cocktail pick. Dip grapes in slightly beaten egg, then roll in Equal.

Ingredients One Serving

White unsweetened grape juice	1/2 cup
Bitters	1-2 dashes
Lemon juice	1/4 tsp
Equal	1-2 packets
Club soda	1/3 cup

Stir first 4 ingredients together in wine glass. Add club soda and enough ice to fill glass. 92 calories per 6-ounce serving, 2 fruits.

Frozen Mockarita — GDS

Ingredients One Serving

Cold water	1/2 cup
Lemon juice	1/4 cup
Lime juice	2 tbl
Equal	4-5 packets
Ice	4-6 cubes

Combine all ingredients in blender. Blend on high for 10 seconds, or until slushy. If desired, salt rim of cocktail glass before filling. 50 calories per 8-ounce serving, 1 fruit.

Equal Nog — GDS

Ingredients for Eight Servings

1 cup nonfat dry milk powder	24 packets Equal
1/2 tsp rum extract	2 cups skim milk
1/2 cup warm water	1 tsp brandy extract
2 eggs	1/2 tsp nutmeg

Combine first 3 ingredients in blender. Blend on high for 5-10 minutes or until smooth and creamy. Add extracts and eggs; blend until well-mixed. Add skim milk and blend until smooth and creamy. Refrigerate until chilled. Pour into punch cups and sprinkle with nutmeg. Use within 4 days. Makes eight 4-ounces servings, each with 110 calories and each equalling 1 nonfat milk.

Amaretto Cocoa – GDS

Garnish with low-calorie whipped topping and toasted, slivered almonds.

Ingredients One Serving

Skim milk	1 cup
Unsweetened cocoa powder	1 tbl
Equal	1-2 packets
Almond extract	$1/8$ tsp

Heat milk on low in saucepan. Combine cocoa, Equal and almond extract in mug. Gradually stir in hot milk. Serve immediately. 110 calories per 8-ounce serving, 1 nonfat milk.

Minty Cocoa – GDS

Follow Amaretto Cocoa recipe, but substitute mint extract for almond. Add an extra drop or two if you prefer a mintier flavor. Use mint extract sparingly though – a little goes a long way.

Mocha Cocoa – GDS

Follow Amaretto Cocoa recipe, but replace almond extract with one tablespoon (tbl) instant coffee powder or crystals (decaffeinated if desired) for each serving. This recipe and the Minty Cocoa each have the same calories as the Amaretto Cocoa and equal 1 nonfat milk.

Hot Sherry Tea – GDS

This is good to take to football games. It is essentially a free drink with only 15 calories per 8-ounce serving.

Ingredients per Four Servings

Unsweetened instant ice tea powder	2 tbl
Boiling water	4 cups
Lemon juice	3 tbl
Sherry extract	4 tsp
Equal	y-8 packets

Nog   Combine instant tea and boiling water in pitcher, or used brewed tea. Stir in rest of ingredients. Pour into four mugs.

Hot Orange Gold Rush – GDS

Ingredients per Four Servings

Unsweetened orange juice	4 cups
Almond extract	$1/2$ tsp
Equal	4-8 packets

Heat orange juice in saucepan. Remove from heat; add almond extract and Equal. Pour into four mugs and serve immediately. 130 calories per 8-ounce serving, 2 fruits.

The Basic Shasta Shake — SB

1 (12-oz) can Diet Shasta (any flavor)
$^1/_3$ cup instant nonfat dry milk
1 portion fresh fruit*
$^1/_8$ tsp vanilla extract
Salt to taste
$^1/_4$ tsp extract*
1 cup coarsely crushed ice (about 12 cubes)

Combine all ingredients in top of blender. Blend on high until frothy. Makes 1 quart. About 160 calories in all, 1 fruit and 1 nonfat milk.

*Your choice to complement soda flavor used, such as berries, orange, pineapple, or cantaloupe. If you want more fruit in each quart of mixture, account for it in your daily diet calculations.

Velvet Vanilla Creme — SB

1 can Diet Shasta Creme Soda
$^3/_4$ cup instant nonfat dry milk
2 tsp vanilla extract
1 dash salt

Blend all ingredients together on high. Serve well chilled. Each of the three 8-ounce servings has 90 calories, 1 nonfat milk.

SOUPS

Fresh Tomato and Bean Soup — CPC

$^1/_2$ cup navy beans
$1^1/_2$ pounds tomatoes, peeled, cored, and chopped
$3^1/_2$ cups water, divided
1 tablespoon vegetable oil
$^1/_4$ tsp Sweet'n Low Liquid sugar substitute
$^1/_2$ cup chopped celery
$^1/_3$ cup chopped onion
$^1/_2$ tsp Italian seasoning, crushed
2 cloves garlic, minced, crushed
$^1/_2$ tsp salt
$^1/_4$ tsp thyme, crushed
$^1/_8$ tsp pepper

In saucepan, combine beans and 2 cups water; bring to a boil. Simmer about 2 minutes. Cover; set aside about 1 hour. Add additional water to saucepan to make 2 cups. Cover; simmer about $1^1/_2$ hours.

About 30 minutes before end of cooking time, in saucepan in hot oil, cook and stir celery, onion, and garlic about 4 minutes. Add tomatoes, Sweet'n Low sugar substitute, Italian seasoning, salt, thyme, pepper, and remaining water. Bring to a boil. Cover; simmer about 20 minutes. Drain beans; add to tomato mixture. Cover; simmer about 5 minutes. Makes 6 1-cup servings, each with 110 calories, 1 bread-starch and 1 cooked vegetable. Negligible fat. You may have one helping of this soup a day, as a substitute for one slice of Malsovit bread.

Borscht — CPC

2 8³/₄-ounce cans julienne beets
10 drops Sweet'n Low Liquid
1 tbl vegetable oil
¹/₂ tsp dill weed
¹/₄ cup chopped onion
¹/₈ tsp pepper
1 cup shredded cabbage
¹/₄ cup plain low-fat yogurt
1 cup beef broth
1 tbl cider vinegar

In food processor or blender, puree 1 can beets; set aside. In saucepan in hot oil, cook onion about 3 minutes. Add cabbage; cook about 8-10 minutes. Add beef broth, pureed beets, julienne beets, vinegar, Sweet'n Low liquid, dill weed and pepper; bring to a boil. Cover; simmer about 20 minutes. Serve hot or chilled, topped with yogurt. Makes four ³/₄-cup servings, each with 95 calories, 2 cooked vegetables, negligible fat and lowfat milk.

BAKED GOODS

Oat Bran Muffins — GDS

Ingredients
1¹/₂ cups low-sugar bran cereal crumbs*
5 packets Equal
¹/₂ cup raisins
1 tablespoon baking powder
1 cup skim milk
2 eggs beaten
1 tablespoon oil
2 tablespoons Mott's unsweetened apple sauce
*Use half low-sugar bran cereal with NutraSweet and half oat bran cereal.

Line microwave muffin pan with paper baking cups. Crush cereal and combine dry ingredients. In a separate bowl, combine moist ingredients. Mix dry and moist ingredients, let stand for about 5 minutes. Stir. Fill muffin cups ³/₄ full. Microwave on medium (50%) for 6 minutes. Each of the 10 muffins produced has about 110 calories, 1 bread-starch and ¹/₂ fat portions. One muffin a day is allowed, replacing one of the slices of Malsovit bread required.

Other muffin recipes may be obtained from Quaker Oats Company, or by reading the *8-Week Cholesterol Cure*, by Robert E. Kowalski (Harper & Row).

Most bran muffins are equal to 1 bread-starch and $^1/_2$ fat portions, just like the above recipe.

SALADS

Molded Perfection Salad – GDS

1 envelope unflavored gelatin
$^1/_2$ cup minced celery
$^1/_4$ cup cold water
$^1/_2$ cup shredded red cabbage
$^1/_2$ cups unsweetened orange juice
$^1/_2$ cup shredded green cabbage
12 packets Equal
1 tbl minced chives
$1^1/_4$ cups shredded carrot

In small saucepan, sprinkle gelatin over cold water. Let stand 1 minute. Heat, stirring constantly until gelatin dissolves. Remove from heat, stir in orange juice and Equal. Chill about 25 minutes or until slightly thickened. Stir in vegetables and chives. Pour into 1-quart mold, sprayed with non-stick coating; chill about 4 hours, or until set. Unmold to serve. Makes 8 $^1/_2$-cup servings, each with 41 calories, $^1/_2$ fruit portion. Could be used as a snack between meals, or as part of a meal.

Yogurt Cucumber Salad – GDS

1 medium cucumber, thinly sliced
4 packets Equal
$^1/_2$ cup thinly sliced red onions
$^1/_2$ tsp salt
$^1/_2$ cup plain lowfat yogurt
$^1/_8$ tsp pepper

Combine cucumber and onion slices in a bowl. Combine remaining ingredients and pour over slices. Toss. Serve immediately. Each of the $4^1/_2$ cup servings has 36 calories and may be considered as a free food if only one is eaten. If two servings, count as one vegetable.

Crisp Sweet Slaw – GDS

Slaw:
4 cups shredded cabbage
1 cup chopped green pepper
$^1/_2$ cup chopped onion.

Dressing:
$^1/_4$ cup cider vinegar
1 tsp celery seed
$^1/_2$ cup apple juice or cider

1 tsp dry mustard
3 tbl vegetable oil
1 tsp salt
8 packets Equal
$\frac{1}{8}$ tsp pepper

Combine slaw ingredients. Whisk together dressing ingredients. Pour over slaw, toss to blend. Refrigerate until served. Each of the eight $\frac{1}{2}$-cup servings has 75 calories, 1 fat and 1 free vegetable if only one serving used.

SOURCES FOR RECIPE INFORMATION

Write the companies at the addresses given below, or look on your grocery shelves for offers on the packages of Sweet'n Low and Equal.

GDS – G.D. Searle Company's NutraSweet or Equal
Equal Consumer Affairs,
Box 8517,
Chicago, Illinois 60680

SB – Shasta Beverages,
26901 Industrial Blvd.,
Hayward CA 94545

CPC – Cumberland Packing Corp.
Dept HHR
60 Flushing Avenue
Brooklyn, NY 11205

If you are worried about the safety of artificial sweeteners, remember that most of the bad publicity about them is generated by people who receive grants from the sugar industry. No wonder they find all these allegedly horrible problems with artificial sweetener use! For a balanced viewpoint, write the Calorie Control Council at the address given at the beginning of this appendix.

APPENDIX FOUR

BARIATRICS, THE NEWEST SPECIALTY

Bariatrics is one of the most fascinating of all the medical disciplines. Derived from the Greek word, *baros* (weight), the word for medical management of obesity was coined by Dr. Raymond Ellis Dietz of Harrisburg, Pennsylvania over 25 years ago. Dr. Dietz, one of the pioneers of Bariatrics, still practices this specialty, along with over 500 other physicians in this country.

A bariatrician is a physician who specializes completely, or partly, in the medical management of obesity. He or she draws on many disciplines of medicine, including internal medicine, psychiatry, and endocrinology. Extensive knowledge of pharmacology, biochemistry, physiology, pathology, and psychology are required, particularly for the doctors who are board-certified by the American Society of Bariatric Physicians.

Almost every major city has at least one bariatrician, or member of the bariatric society listed here. In order to be a member of the society, a doctor must demonstrate that he or she conforms to good medical practices best illustrated by the Standards of Practice of the American Society of Bariatric Physicians. Those conforming to these Standards will prominently display a plaque to that effect in their offices.

It pays to use someone who is thoroughly grounded in the latest techniques of weight reduction and who will take your problems seriously. An unsympathetic physician is the last thing a person with a weight problem needs. Avoid the clods in white coats who tell you to "just push away from the table."

You are better off with your own personal physician than with someone poorly trained and poorly motivated to provide you with the proper care. Especially avoid the "hole in the wall" lay clinics that try to con you into paying thousands of dollars, usually in advance, for some dubious method. There has been a steady stream of victims who have reported their problems to the Georgia Department of Consumer Affairs, usually too late, and Georgia is not the only state afflicted with these crooks. While it is true that there are a few excellent lay-run organizations around, too large a proportion of them are fly-by-night and run by former spa managers with little or no knowledge, except that needed to separate you from your money with high pressure sales tactics.

The so-called "fat doctors" with their amphetamine mills are rapidly fading away, but a few are still around. Make sure your doctor is a member of his county and state medical societies. Check with his county society to see if he has any complaints filed against him. In the case of a lay clinic, check with your local Better Business Bureau or your state Department of Consumer Affairs.

For those of you who wish to have your physician refer you to a bariatrician, you may write or call the society listed below. The information is free, but a self-addressed, stamped envelope enclosed with your request will expedite the return of information on bariatricians in your local area.

The American Society of Bariatric Physicians
5600 S. Quebec St.
Suite 160-D
Englewood, Colorado 80111
(303) 779-4833
Mr. James Merker, Executive Director